HEADW

HERBALISM

Frances Büning   Paul Hambly

Headway · Hodder & Stoughton

For Eleanor, whose love of life is a joy and inspiration

We deeply appreciate the enormous amount of help we have had while writing this book, from reading the manuscript and making suggestions to emotional support and baby-sitting. We would like to thank the following people: Rhona Thomas, Nick Beak, Gregory Smith, Charlotte Rolleston-Smith, Nic and Kirsten Rowley, Tina and John James, Lisa Webber, Maya Morgan, Susan Birch, Judy Fraser, Holly Gothard, Jayne Booth, Sue Hart and our parents . . . Thank you all for your care and support.

The authors and Publishers would like to thank: for giving permission to reproduce copyright material in this book, The Ancient Art and Architecture Collection (p. 4), Chelsea Physic Garden (p. 6), J. Allan Cash Photolibrary (p. 24), Fresh Fruit and Vegetable Information Bureau, London (p. 25); for the cover photograph, Christina Jansen and Siobhan Chandler; for all commissioned photographs, Roddy Paine; for the drawings Helen Lavinia Reed.

British Library Cataloguing in Publication Data

Hambly, Paul
  Herbalism. – (Headway Lifeguides)
  I. Title II. Buning, Frances III. Series
  615

ISBN 0–340–56575–6

First published 1993
Impression number   10 9 8 7 6 5 4 3 2 1
Year   1998 1997 1996 1995 1994 1993

© 1993 Frances Büning & Paul Hambly

Typeset by Wearset, Boldon, Tyne and Wear
Printed in Great Britain for the educational publishing division of Hodder & Stoughton Ltd, Mill Road, Dunton Green, Sevenoaks, Kent TN13 2YA by Thomson Litho Ltd.

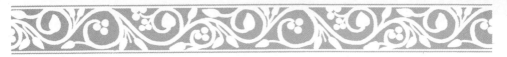

CONTENTS

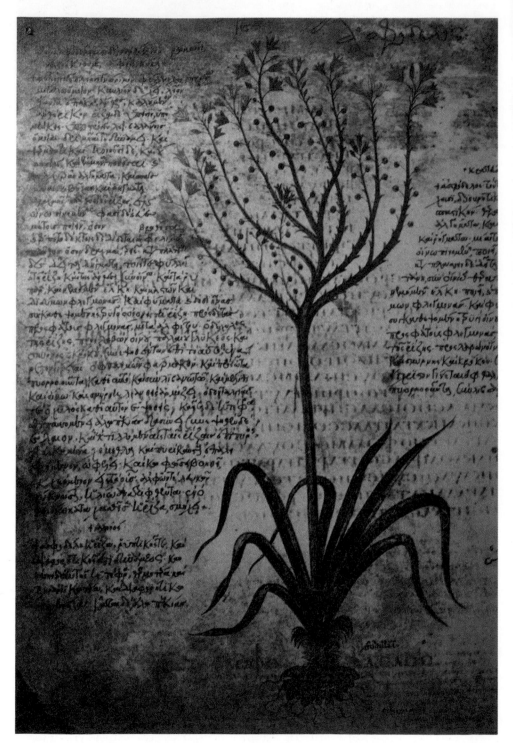

Dioscorides manuscript On materia medica *512 AD, Constantinople*

INTRODUCTION

The medicine of mankind

Herbal medicine is indigenous to all the cultures of the world and has evolved quite independently all over the globe throughout history. Herbs have always been synonymous with medicine and herbal medicine is the oldest form of therapy currently practised by mankind. Indeed, seven of the eight species of plants identified from the grains of pollen found in the grave of Neanderthal man in Iraq, some 60,000 years old, are used by herbalists today; most of the plants recorded in use over the centuries still grow around us and are readily accessible for self-medication.

Plants provide us with nutrients and contain vitamins, minerals, antibiotics and hormonal substances in a form that is easy for the human body to assimilate, fulfilling its requirements as both food and medicine. Moreover, research has now shown that plants have an energy field that can be likened to the magnetic field that surrounds the human body. It makes much more sense to use natural, organic material that has life and is in harmony with man than a synthetic, lifeless material which cannot enhance the life force.

> **66** *It presents itself as a gift of nature, with a cosmic naturalness that makes it the obvious choice for a first treatment approach. Generations have made use of it, gained experience, and cherished it, like a historical treasure, as a source of therapy.* **99**
> Professor H E Bock, *Herbal Medicine.*

The green revolution

For many years, an increasing number of people have become dissatisfied with orthodox medicine and moved towards alternative ways of healing. This is part of a wider awareness not just of our health but of our environment and our responsibility to the planet.

By incorporating herbal medicine into our lives in favour of synthetic medicine we can help to reduce the pollution of our planet and save the lives of countless laboratory animals. Moreover, there is no doubt that the employment of herbs in favour of synthesised drugs would save millions of pounds on drug expenditure. It is, however, impossible for drug companies to patent a plant and so there is resistance to this sort of change.

It is very difficult to analyse plants' medicinal properties exactly, especially those without very powerful actions, as there is usually an array of active constituents. We need to see a move away from the quest to isolate plant principles towards the development of assessing the whole plant and its medicinal action as endowed by nature.

Today we see the application of science to empirical knowledge. Modern methods confirm the actions of a plant that has been used successfully for centuries. Science can play an important role in plant medicines, including standardisation and quality control. Let us hope to see the best of both worlds merge and go forward together.

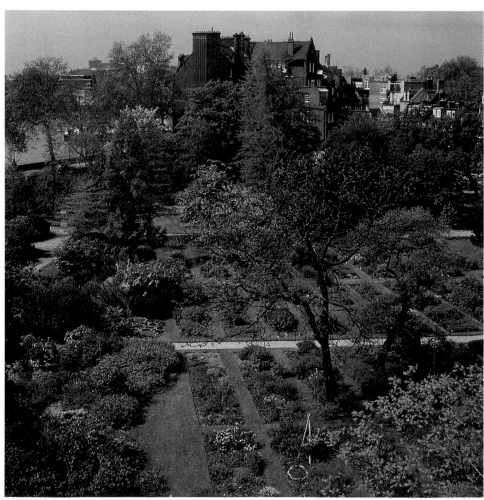

View from Swan Walk, Chelsea Physic Garden

How to use this book

Our purpose has been to simplify the information available and to outline the principles of using herbal medicine as part of a holistic treatment.

We suggest you acquaint yourself thoroughly with *The principles and practice of herbal medicine* (page 8) and *How to survive modern living* (page 23) for a thorough grounding to the book.

The ailments specifically discussed in this book are arranged alphabetically in *An A–Z of ailments*, on page 62. Each entry starts with a brief description and diagnosis, followed by sections which give advice on when to seek professional help, exercise, diet and supplements, herbs and finally, commercially available products. Refer to *The natural pharmacy* on page 16 for how to prepare the herbs.

If your condition is one which needs a major long-term change (more than one month) to diet, or you are pregnant or the patient is a child, it is best to seek professional help. Vitamin and mineral supplementation should be reviewed after three months, and should not be taken day-in day-out, unless prescribed by your practitioner.

Although most of the herbs in this book are quite safe to take for long periods of time, it is inadvisable to remain on the same herbs for an extended length of time without consulting a medical herbalist. It is not only that certain herbs, such as the astringents which are commonly used in diarrhoea and colitis, can interfere with absorption of nutrients from the gut if taken inappropriately, but everything changes in time, and whereas one herb was appropriate three months ago, something else might be more suitable now.

> 66 *The study of plant life teaches us to see Man as part of Nature, subject to her laws . . . The more we try and control Nature, instead of using our rightful place within her, the sooner we become aware that we have gone beyond the limit.* 99
> Weiss

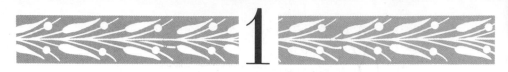

1

THE PRINCIPLES AND PRACTICE OF HERBAL MEDICINE

What is good health?

Health is a positive state which we can build on every day by respecting our needs. This means paying attention to diet, exercise, environment and relaxation. However, the requirements of each individual are different. (For example, some people naturally need more sleep than others.) Health is about learning to accept and respect our limitations.

Learning how to accept and deal with change is also fundamental to our well-being. Change is a state of flow and movement. As soon as we try to stop the flow we go against nature and run into trouble. Fear sets up a negative and static state which resists change, and can be a difficult obstacle to overcome.

Indeed, many sick people are afraid of becoming well because they feel protected from the outside world and secure with their illness. For others, illness is a cry for help, and love. Being well involves taking control, confronting and dealing with life's problems.

How to view disease

Dis-ease is a sign of imbalance and disharmony in the body. It tends to manifest itself when we have overstretched ourselves and have not listened to our body's warnings or when we resist and cannot cope with change. A change of job, moving house, bereavement or any emotional crisis needs to be processed, assimilated and digested by the body in order to move on. This takes time.

Disease is an opportunity to learn about ourselves, to accept our limitations and strengthen our weaknesses. It is easy to hate disease, as if it has been willed upon us from outside, or feel that we deserve to be ill because we are not good enough or have done something terrible. In effect, by hating it, we are hating ourselves, as the illness is a manifestation of part of our being.

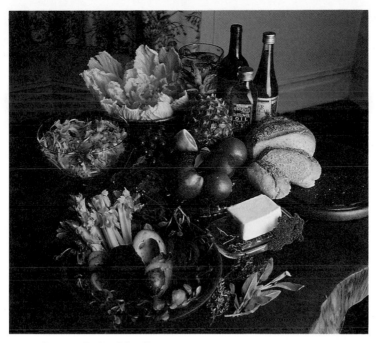

Some basics of a healthy diet

Working preventatively

Your overall aim should be to prevent illness by observing what is outlined above and in *How to survive modern living* on page 23, as well as strengthening the weak areas of your body.

If, and when, illness does occur, the aim is to minimise the severity and length of the condition by enhancing your body's own defences. (For instance, garlic and cider vinegar can be incorporated into your daily diet to protect against infection, particularly during the times of year you tend to be more susceptible to illness.)

Everything you do and consume can have a positive or negative effect on your health. See yourself as building up credits eating good food and taking sufficient exercise, rest and relaxation.

Arriving at a diagnosis

The correct diagnosis is crucial in order to have the right treatment for your problem. Often, you will already have been offered a diagnosis by your doctor. However, apart from identifying the complaint, diagnosis involves deducing which bodily system/s and organs are under strain and need help and whether the condition is caused by infection.

On a physical level, if there are signs of illness, check the temperature of the body. Are the glands swollen, is there pain, loss of appetite, skin rash, diarrhoea? Is the onset of the condition sudden or progressive?

As well as noting the immediate physical symptoms, it is vital to assess the events prior to the problem manifesting itself. It is helpful to write possible contributory events down in chronological order, including accidents, innoculations, travel, the breakdown of a relationship, bereavements and job changes. Note any patterns. Life events are highly important to health.

It can be difficult to assess the situation objectively when you are treating yourself or someone close to you, but at the same time you will be far more aware than an outsider of subtle changes and instinctively know when something is wrong.

When viewing an illness, try to see the person in the context of their whole life, emotions, work, home, relationships. What type of person are they? Have they fulfilled their desires in life, are they rigid in thought, are they very sensitive to criticism, etc? Tension can often be the cause of headaches, constipation or insomnia. In this case, the mind is behind the physical problem but equally, constipation can cause poor concentration. A recurring sore throat might be connected with difficulty in communicating, arthritis an inability to be flexible in daily life. These aspects of an illness should be approached in order to address the situation fully.

With acute problems, such as sore throats and burns, one treats the symptoms and heals the tissues, but with chronic ailments, such as rheumatism or migraine, a wider strategy has to be employed. One can only assess the state of the body by looking at its current symptoms and what has happened to it in the past.

If the illness is of sudden onset, if there is loss of weight, a sudden change in bowel habit, any lumps or growths, or simply no change in the condition despite treatment, it is important to consult your practitioner.

The basic approach to treatment

66 *A good physician practises common sense with a few tools to aid* 99
the process.

Talking is a powerful healer in itself; it always helps to talk about something instead of keeping it bottled up inside. Touch is also important; shaking hands, sharing a hug, giving or having a massage. These simple actions help to give reassurance and encouragement.

Start with using the least intervention and gentlest remedies, but at the same time know when to act. This means using the art of conversation, diet and herbs in the first instance rather than the last resort, reserving drugs and surgery for life-threatening conditions, and as a short-term measure only.

As well as assessing the effect of the mind on the body and determining which system or organ is under strain, you must look at the blood supply. Are the tissues being supplied with nutrients and being cleared of toxins? Are the toxins being eliminated from the body via the kidneys and bowels? How high are energy levels? Is the constitution strong or frail?

Constitution

This varies enormously and has much to do with what you have been handed down from previous generations. If you have indigestion, are frail and prone to tiredness, you will need gentle and restorative herbs along with appropriate dietary changes. If you have indigestion, are always on the go and sleep very little, you will need a calming prescription of completely different herbs.

Circulation

It is important to assess whether you are hot or cold. Do you always have cold hands or feet or do you get hot and sweat easily? The former suggests congestion and poor flow of blood and energy through the body, and circulatory herbs, like **cayenne**, **garlic**, **ginger** and **horseradish**, should be included in your diet and combined with other appropriate herbs. In the latter, the bitters, which are cooling, improve the function of the digestive organs and help to drain toxins out of the system, might be suggested.

Elimination

Pollution from our environment and food builds up in our bodies, especially in the fat tissue and joints. Illness can result, as the body attempts to clean itself. Or the toxins themselves can be an irritant to the system, stressing the immune system and lowering resistance to disease.

The obvious organs of elimination are the bowels and the kidneys, but the lungs, skin and lymphatic system (see below) also play their part. In women, the menstrual cycle is another eliminatory route.

The liver is the power-house and detoxifying organ of the body, dealing with the breakdown of the waste products of digestion. These include food additives, pesticides, hormones, drugs, chemicals and dead bacteria.

Assess whether all the channels are functioning properly. If they are not, toxins will tend to accumulate in the system. Constipation, lymphatic congestion or weak kidneys can all cause skin problems like boils, eczema and psoriasis. Where the system is congested with toxins, the function of these organs can be enhanced by using herbs. Appropriate herbs include **dandelion root** for the liver, **celery seeds** to stimulate the elimination of toxins via the kidneys, **burdock root** to cleanse the tissues and **cleavers** to purify the lymphatic system. Cleansing the system is vital to restore and maintain good health. Diet is fundamental in this. See page 25 in *How to survive modern living*.

Fasting

Fasting can be a very effective way of cleansing and detoxifying the system. When we are ill, especially with a fever, we tend to fast naturally, due to lack of appetite. The body works more efficiently when the digestive system is shut down and attention can be concentrated on dealing with the infection. However, we tend to be very thirsty at these times and it is important to drink plenty of fluids to flush the toxins (from the breakdown of the invading organism) out of the system.

Care needs to be taken when fasting is undertaken as part of therapy. Check with your practitioner that it is appropriate for you. If you are diabetic, suffer from hypoglycaemia, heart problems, cancer, are on any medication, or in poor health, fasting should only be undertaken on the advice of your practitioner. Do not fast if you are pregnant.

If you have never fasted before, choose just one, or, if possible, three days when you can take things quietly. Try to eat sensibly before you go into the fast and when you come out. Choose one fruit, preferably organic, to fast on (white grapes are ideal, but you could eat apples or pears). Eat as much as you want of your chosen fruit, at regular intervals. This means you will be eating several pounds of grapes a day! Alternatively, have some, or all of the fruit as juice. Drink pure water only. Do not fast on water alone, especially if you have never fasted before, as the tendency with water fasts is to throw all the toxins out into the system very quickly, causing great discomfort. Fasting can cause headaches, dizziness and a general feeling of being unwell. This is likely to pass, but if it becomes too uncomfortable, start eating again. (Wholegrain rice will help to rid the system of toxins.) If you suffer from allergies, it is better to fast on vegetable juices, choosing from beetroot, carrot and celery.

Enemas can be a useful adjunct to a fast, especially where there are impacted faeces which are a source of toxins returning to the system. Ask your practitioner about these.

Epsom salt baths ($\frac{1}{2}$ kg per bath), salt rubs and saunas are further useful aids to the cleansing process, but should be undertaken between, not during, fasts, and again, not if you are in poor health.

The immune system

The immune system is vital to good health, protecting us from organisms and clearing up debris from the bodily processes.

The effectiveness of the immune system can be compromised by a number of things: antibiotics, steroids, stress, the contraceptive pill, bereavement, a focus of infection in the body, a poor diet, nutritional deficiency, pollution, genetic factors and smoking. If your immunity is compromised, then problems such as colds, 'flu, swollen glands, or worse, keep returning and depleting you further.

The blood contains cells to attack and destroy organisms. However, the lymphatic system comes into action when the invasion is more severe. This is a network of tiny vessels which carry the fluid lymph. The lymph picks up debris and microbes and carries them via the vessels to the lymph nodes, some of the main sites of immune activity in the body.

The lymph nodes are situated in groups along the main lymphatic channels in the body – the neck, armpits, groin, chest and abdomen. They enlarge when the body is under attack, as they are producing more white blood cells. These groups of lymph nodes are known as the *lymph glands* and can be felt as swollen and tender masses when fighting an infection. They contain large numbers of white blood cells which literally eat up the invading organisms. In a highly infectious disease, antibodies are produced against the organism. These form protection against reinfection with the disease in the future. The liver, spleen, tonsils, adenoids and lining of the small intestine all contain lymphatic tissue. The debris resulting from the infection is carried to the liver to be detoxified and excreted.

A healthy diet is vital for a healthy immune system (please refer to *How to survive modern living* on page 25). Beetroot (which increases cell respiration), garlic and vitamin C, which can be obtained from fresh, raw fruits and vegetables, and the herb **echinacea** all boost the function of the immune system.

Exercise activates what is called the *lymphatic pump*, improving the circulation of lymph around the body and the drainage and elimination of debris.

A good immune system demonstrates that your body is well-balanced and prepares you to deal quickly and effectively with any invading organisms.

Auto-immune disease occurs when the immune system starts to attack the body's own tissues, as in rheumatoid arthritis, for example. When an auto-immune reaction occurs, the control mechanism which normally stops invading organisms has broken down.

Convalescence

We tend to think of convalescence as something for the elderly and infirm but it is something that everyone can benefit from after an illness, when the body needs time to recover and regenerate. This is rarely respected these days when the pace of living is fast. As we have already seen, disease is a sign of imbalance or distress. If we acknowledge this in the early stages and take time to deal with it, the problem takes less time to clear up. The body takes time to heal and nature will not be hurried.

Rest and good nutrition are both required. Fruit and vegetable juices are easily absorbed and digested.

Fresh air and gentle exercise, when possible, are vital. Get the limbs moving as much as you can to start the strengthening process and get the blood flowing.

Appetite and digestive function can be poor after an illness, but the following can help to speed recovery:

- Angostura or Swedish bitters or **dandelion root** help to stimulate the digestive system.
- **Angelica**, which is a warming digestive tonic and **centaury** are gentle restorative herbs.
- Porridge, artichoke and alfalfa are excellent foods for convalescence.
- Have plenty of fresh, raw fruit and vegetables especially apricots, parsley, spinach and grapes.
- **Slippery elm** and Spirulina are very nutritive, particularly where appetite and digestion are poor.
- Brewer's yeast and **kelp** supply extra vitamins.
- Take vitamin C and Floradix liquid or tablets.
- **Nettles** are high in vitamins and minerals, especially iron.
- **Hawthorn** can be used where the heart has been put under a lot of strain.
- **Borage** and **liquorice** both help to restore the function of the adrenal glands which are put under strain during times of illness.
- **Vervain** is a tonic and restorative to the whole system.
- Add a little **ginger** to your herbs.
- **Ginseng** can be a very useful restorative. However it should never be taken during acute illness. It has a hormonal action so can affect the menstrual cycle. It should only be taken for a month at a time.

Using herbs

Herbs work on a physical level, interacting physiologically in the body's chemistry; they also work on a more subtle level, releasing mental blockages, thereby restoring the balance between mind and body.

Herbs can be used as soon as a problem appears, without waiting for the outcome of complicated tests. They support the body and restore function without blocking a specific pathway or enzyme. They can be used alongside orthodox drugs, but it is best to consult a medical herbalist about this.

With practice, you can use herbs successfully to treat many health problems. It is, however important to remember that taking responsibility for your health also means being able to recognise when you need professional advice.

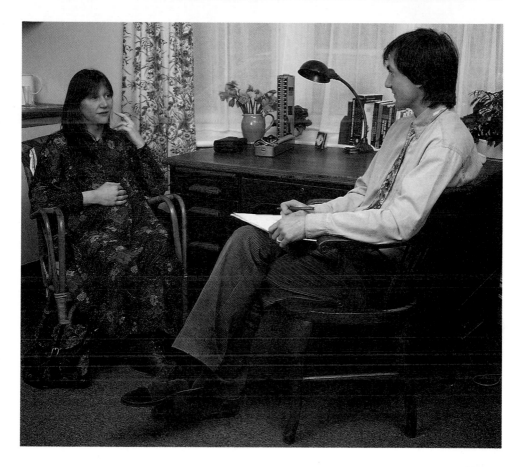

Consulting a medical herbalist

It is a good idea to get to know a medical herbalist in your area. An initial consultation is important to assess your medical history as well as any present health problems. It is also the time to decide whether this is the right practitioner for you. Nothing can replace a consultation. It is extremely unreliable to try to diagnose over the phone or by letter. However, once they know you, and perhaps your family, most herbalists are quite happy to give advice over the telephone.

A consultation will involve looking into your past medical history. This may seem unrelated to your present situation, but it often uncovers a clue to what is happening at the present time, with past and present illnesses creating a pattern. A physical examination, such as taking your blood pressure or listening to your chest, might also be necessary.

Diagnosis results in the prescription of individually tailored medicine, which can vary widely from one individual to the next, even if they are suffering from similar problems. The person is more important than the disease.

2

THE NATURAL PHARMACY

How to use the herbs

Herbs can be used in a great variety of ways, depending on the herbs themselves and the form of treatment most suitable for a particular condition.

Infusions/teas

These are made using the leaves, flowers or aerial parts of the fresh or dried herb.

The process is like making ordinary, loose-leaf tea. Put 1 tsp of the dried or 2 tsp of the fresh herb in a teapot. Add a cup of boiling water and brew for 10 to 15 minutes before straining.

The standard dose is 1 tsp per cup 3 times a day.

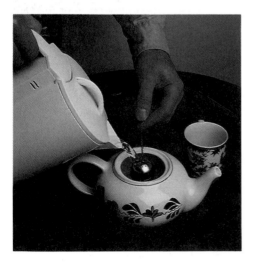

Decoctions

These are made from the woodier parts of herbs – roots, bark and seeds – which need to be simmered to extract the active ingredients.

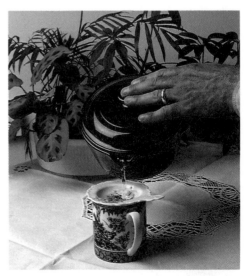

The material should be cut or crushed into small pieces in order to gain the best extraction. Use a stainless steel, enamelled or glass saucepan with a lid, as aluminium can combine with some of the herbs. Simmer for 10 to 15 minutes.

Use in the same dosage as an infusion, but allow a little more water.

Capsules and tablets

Capsules can be made up at home using powdered herbs. Grind the herb to a powder in a coffee grinder or pestle and mortar. The standard size capsule is 00 and 2 of these are equivalent to 1 tsp of tincture or an infusion using 2 tsp of herb per cup. A standard dose is 2 capsules 3 times a day.

The capsules should be separated, keeping the two different parts in different piles. Either by hand, or using a capsule maker, pack the larger part of the capsule with the powder then push the smaller top section on firmly.

A simple and inexpensive capsule-making machine is available from *East West Herbs*, see page 159. See page 160 for suppliers of gelatine and non-animal capsules.

Capsules and tablets are useful when taking strong-tasting herbs. However, bitter herbs begin their work as soon as they reach the taste buds and really do need to be tasted.

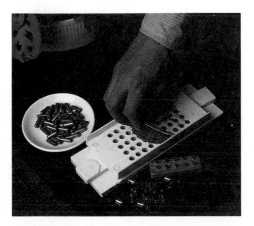

Tinctures

These are concentrated extracts of either fresh or dried herbs. A mixture of water and alcohol is used to extract the ingredients in the herb and to preserve them. Different herbs require a different percentage of alcohol in the mixture, depending on the ingredients being extracted. For example, **myrrh** needs a 90 per cent solution in order to extract the resin it contains. Other herbs require the minimum amount of alcohol, which is 25 per cent.

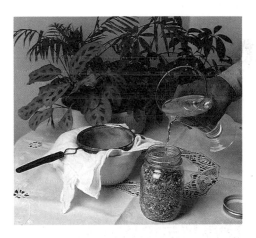

To make up a tincture at home, vodka or brandy, which are equivalent to 45 per cent alcohol, will normally be fine. Use 1 part of dried herb to 5 parts of alcohol, or, if using the fresh plant, 1 part of herb to 2 parts alcohol. For example, place 200 g of dried herb in a large jar and pour over 1 litre of alcohol, close the jar tightly with an airtight lid and store it away from the light. Shake the jar every day, and leave it for at least 2 weeks before straining and squeezing through a muslin bag or simple wine press. Discard the herb, preferably on to the compost heap, and store the liquid in a dark bottle.

Tinctures will keep well for 2 to 3 years.

The standard dose is 1 tsp 3 times a day for most herbs.

Contraindications   Tinctures should not be used if you have an allergy to alcohol, have an alcohol problem or suffer from liver disease.

Syrups

Tincture, tea or fresh material is used to make syrup with brown sugar, honey or concentrated apple juice. An onion, for example, can be cut, placed in an airtight container, and covered with brown sugar or honey. Leave in a warm place overnight and then strain. Store in an airtight container. Syrups are an excellent way of disguising the taste of medicine (especially useful for children) as well as being medicinal in themselves.

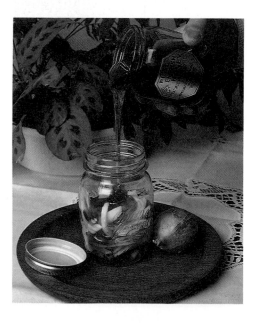

Baths

These are an excellent way of administering herbs to babies and young children since the skin is a very good medium through which to absorb the herbs into the system.

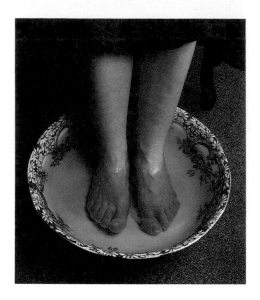

The herbs are made up in the same way as infusions and decoctions but using 2 tablespoons of material. Once the tea has been strained into the bath or footbath, more boiling water can be poured on to the residual material and brewed again before straining into the bath. Stay in the water for 8 to 10 minutes.

Eyebaths

These are prepared in the same way as an infusion. Simmer for 1 or 2 minutes to achieve sterility, then strain through muslin or a coffee filter. The addition of a few grains of salt to the eyebath is helpful.

Alternatively, add 1 to 3 drops of tincture to an eyebathful of distilled water.

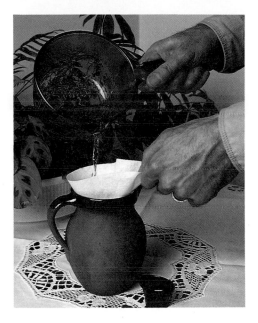

your chosen oil then screw the lid on tightly. Place it in a window for a minimum of 2 weeks. The oil turns dark red when finally ready. Strain through muslin and store in a closed jar. **Marigolds** can be similarly infused. Green leafy material such as **comfrey** leaf and stems should be infused in the dark.

The oils have good keeping qualities and readily accept the addition of essential oils.

Garlic oil

Take a whole bulb of **garlic**. Peel and crush each clove, place in a jar, cover in a cold-pressed oil and seal. The oil may be used within 24 hours but the longer you leave it, the stronger it becomes. Strain when you feel it is ready and keep in an airtight container.

Herbal oils or fixed oils

These are made by steeping the flowers, leaves or aerial parts of the plant in vegetable oil, such as sunflower or, preferably, cold-pressed olive oil.

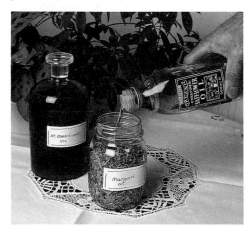

To make **St John's wort** oil, for example, take a screw-top glass jar and pack it with the clean, freshly picked flowers. Fill to the brim with

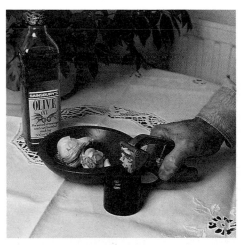

Essential oils

These potent healing substances can be viewed as a concentration of the whole plant, the macrocosm within the microcosm. They can be used effectively in massage oil (1 to

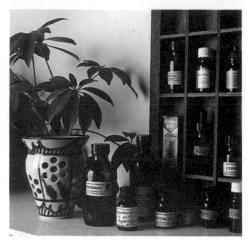

2 drops per ml of a base oil), baths (10 drops per bath), or ointments (1 drop per 10 ml). They should only be taken internally if advised by a qualified practitioner. They can only be made by specialists.

Creams and ointments

One of the easiest ways to make up your own cream is to obtain an aqueous base cream from a chemist and add your own ingredients. This cream will take water- or oil-based products, so you can add teas, infusions, decoctions, fixed oils, essential oils or even powdered dried herbs.

Ointments are made by taking a fixed oil such as **comfrey** or **marigold** and adding beeswax. Both need to be gently warmed in order to mix them together. Surprisingly little beeswax is required. To test, dip a spoon into the mixture and cool it off to room temperature. If it makes a mass yet easily spreads over the skin, you have used the right proportions. Pour into screw-top jars. The addition of a few drops of essential oil (such as **tea tree**) will improve its keeping qualities.

Compresses

Compresses are simply cold teas, decoctions or tinctures poured on to a suitable piece of cloth, for example, a piece of muslin or a handkerchief, and applied to the skin over the affected area.

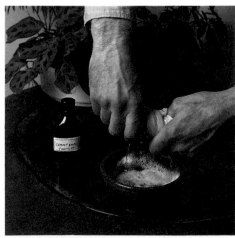

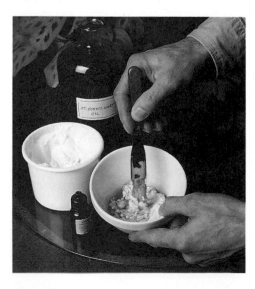

Poultices

Poultices are packs of herb applied to the body. Find a cotton or muslin bag large enough to cover the part of the body being treated. Take the mixture of herbs required and add the same volume of powdered **slippery elm** or other carrier, such as potato powder. Place 1 to 4 tablespoons of this mix in the bag. Slowly pour boiling water into the bag in order to thoroughly wet the contents. It will gradually absorb more water over the next 5 minutes. You want to aim to have a mix that is wet yet not dripping, as it has to stay in place for 15 minutes. As soon as the poultice has cooled sufficiently, apply it to the skin and leave it there till cool.

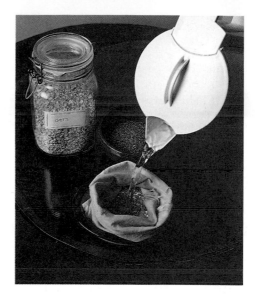

Dosages

Recommendations on dosages for single herbs are given throughout the book. However, where none is mentioned, apply the standard dose as given above. Standard doses can generally be doubled during acute illness, such as 'flu.

As most medicine needs to be individually tailored, you will find you need to make mixtures of the different herbs. This means that you mix the herbs first in the right proportions then apply the standard dose, not that you take each herb separately at the standard dose. As an example, for a headache, you might choose **skullcap**, **wood betony** and **lavender**. The suggested dosage for all of these is 1 to 2 tsp per cup. Since you are making a mixture of them, combine 1 part of each herb, for example 1 oz of each, and use 1 to 2 tsp per cup of this mixture.

When there is a choice between using 1 or 2 tsp per cup, start with the lower amount and increase to the higher amount if the effect is not strong enough or if the symptoms are severe. This also applies to the number of times a day you take the dose.

Body weight also plays a part in dosages. Someone who is slight will need a smaller dose than someone who is tall and heavy.

When the recommendation is to take the herbs *as required*, you can safely take the suggested dose every 3 hours or as sips or drops throughout the day.

The available products are given as an alternative to making up your own medicines.

For dosages for children see page 51.

A basic dispensary

Listed below are the herbs that should be included in a basic medicine chest. They might be stored as tinctures or dried herbs. If they are dried herbs, they should be kept in airtight containers in a cool, dark place and dated.

The shelf-life of dried herbs is about a year (from one harvest to the next), although roots tend to maintain their medicinal properties a little longer. Tinctures will keep for much longer.

For internal use

cayenne	lemon balm
chamomile	limeflowers
dandelion root	peppermint
echinacea	thyme
elderflowers	nettles
eyebright	valerian
ginger	

The Bach Flower Rescue Remedy should also be added to the medicine chest.

For external use

Ointments of arnica, calendula and comfrey, St John's wort oil, distilled witch hazel

Essential oils

Eucalyptus, lavender, tea tree, thyme.

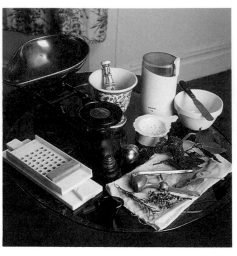

Equipment you will find useful for making up your own herbal remedies at home

Where to obtain your herbs

Talk to your medical herbalist who can advise you on what is most appropriate for your situation. If you have children, for example, there will be some specific remedies to have on hand.

- There is also a list of suppliers at the back of this book. See page 159.

HOW TO SURVIVE MODERN LIVING

The pace of life in the modern western world can only be described as frantic, with a potentially self-destructive striving for material possession. Everything is designed to be quick and convenient. As an extension of this quest for speed and control, we tend to expect instant cures, finding it hard to take time to be ill, let alone to convalesce, ignoring the fact that the body needs time to heal.

Looking back at previous generations, we can see that illnesses have changed. Indeed, there are patterns to disease which have a tendency to ebb and flow, as well as disappear to be replaced by something different. Changes in hygiene are the most obvious cause for the disappearance of many previously life-threatening diseases. The emergence of 'new' diseases like AIDS, Alzheimer's, auto-immune conditions, candidiasis, ME, post-viral syndrome and the increase of cancer suggests, however, a continuing, wider correlation with our changing environment and social attitudes. Modern diseases tend to reflect suppression of the immune system, toxic accumulation and stress, rather than poor living conditions.

It is vital to find ways of coping with the pace of life, take time to regenerate ourselves, in mind, body and spirit, and seek personal fulfilment and well-being.

Pollution in our environment

We are surrounded by many forms of pollution – noise and electromagnetic radiation, as well as the more obvious pollution in the air, water and food. Our lives revolve around electricity, with a host of electrical appliances, television, computers and VDU screens as part of our normal everyday life. These all give off electromagnetic radiation that can interfere with the electromagnetic field of the human body in the susceptible individual.

In the home, synthetic fibres in furniture, bedding and flooring, clothes, and particularly the chemicals used to treat them (to make them fire-retardant, for example) can give off toxic vapours. Household chemicals like bleach, disinfectant, polish and detergents are other hazards, as are the fumes from paints and insulation materials, and

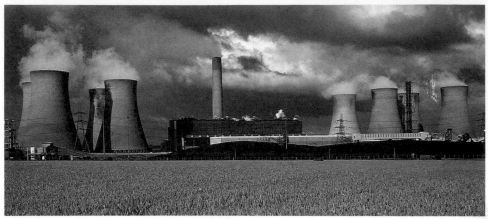

Pollution – the price we pay for modern living

carbon monoxide fumes from gas heaters. Cigarette smoke, fluorescent lighting and air-conditioning add to the very unhealthy and artificial atmosphere in which we live and work.

Some people are more sensitive to these influences than others but there are ways of protecting yourself and enhancing the environment in which you live and work. The use of anti-radiation screens, ionisers, plants, non-fluorescent lighting and air filters can make a significant difference. It is worth changing to more environmentally- and people-friendly products and choosing new items, such as furniture and electrical equipment, with care. The effects rebound on us all in the end.

Orthodox drugs

These play an irrefutable role in the health-care system, notably in acute, life-threatening situations. They are, however, not always appropriate for long-term therapy, or for use in the first instance, when a dietary change, counselling or herbal treatment would be sufficient to cure the condition.

Orthodox drugs work by suppressing symptoms and blocking normal physiological functions. This causes side-effects and provide the body with another source of toxic accumulation.

Antibiotics

Without doubt, antibiotics have a place in the treatment of serious infections and have saved many lives. They are, however, inappropriate for the vast proportion of infections which are self-limiting, and for infections which are more likely to be caused by a virus rather than bacteria, and will not respond to treatment with antibiotics.

In time, the body tends to become immune to the effect of antibiotics, especially when prescribed frequently. Moreover, they tend to drive infections deeper into the system, for example, ear infections which lead to glue ear and sinus trouble in later life. They weaken the immune system and leave the body susceptible to further, repeated infections.

Side-effects include disturbance of the intestinal flora causing thrush (see *Candidiasis*), for example. To prevent the side-effects of antibiotics if you have to take them, eat live yoghurt or take Superdophilus as soon as you start the course of antibiotics. **Garlic**, apple cider vinegar, **dandelion root** and **echinacea** can all be taken to boost the immune system and help elimination of toxins from the drug and the infection.

What is a healthy diet?

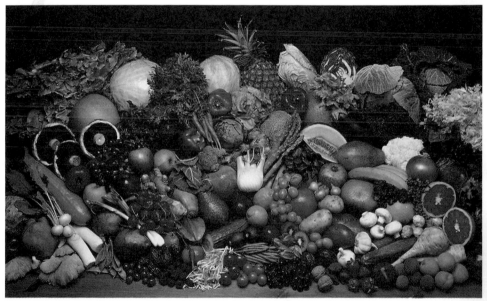

Is our food as good as it looks?

Food is a fundamental ingredient to our well-being and should be thought of as of paramount importance. It is worth paying more for and searching out good quality food as a sound health insurance policy.

However, a healthy diet for one person is not necessarily right for somebody else. Indeed, at different stages of our lives we have different nutritional requirements, depending on age, activity, condition or environment. Try to eat as healthily as possible without becoming paranoid about it. Bear in mind that '*a little* of what you fancy does you good'.

Years ago, we ate a much wider variety of foods, with seasonal variations; today we have tomatoes, oranges, peas etc. all year round. The wide variety of choice on the supermarket shelf is countered by the need for products to survive long enough to be sold. This means that foods like tomatoes are chosen for their ability to travel long distances without being damaged – so those with tougher skins are sold. Growth inhibitors are used to stop potatoes sprouting and fruit, like bananas, is sprayed with ripening agents between its country of origin and destination. Our diets have diminished from a variety of about 2000 different foods throughout a year to about 60, with dairy produce, wheat and eggs predominating in the western diet.

In a world where pollution is rife, it is difficult to know what is actually doing you good. Chemicals find their way into the food chain and build up in concentration. Generally speaking, it is safer to choose foods low on the scale, such as fruit, vegetables, grains and pulses. Meat, fish and dairy products are high up in the food chain and have been shown to contain higher levels of contaminants. These are absorbed into our bodies and can be transferred to a baby via the placenta and breast milk. Some of these chemicals can be very hard to excrete, and with daily exposure, the build-up will eventually cause problems. Agricultural chemical residues tend to be highest in the skins of fruit and vegetables or outer husks of seeds and grains. This makes eating non-organic potato skins and wholegrain bread rather a hazard.

Junk foods, processed foods and soft drinks supply worthless nutrition, tending to be full of sugars and fats, and very high in phosphates. These can lead to lack of absorption of vital nutrients and deprive the body further by utilising precious resources in their metabolism, thereby robbing the body of B vitamins and minerals.

If we eat organically grown foods as much as we can, we are helping ourselves enormously. Organic foods contain higher concentrations of vitamins and minerals than conventional produce and do not contain the cocktail of pesticides, herbicides, fungicides, inorganic fertilizers, growth inhibitors, ripening agents etc. These chemicals combined with food additives, such as colourings, preservatives, anticaking agents, antioxidants, at the very best make our livers and kidneys work harder than they need and at worst cause allergies and hyperactivity, and are strongly associated with cancer formation. Moreover, organic food tastes better and has natural vitality!

Protein

Eggs, fish, meat, milk products, poultry and soya beans are all complete proteins – containing all the essential amino acids. Good sources of non-animal protein, other than soya, are derived from grains, pulses, nuts and seeds. Vegetable proteins (except soya) are incomplete proteins, so need to be eaten in combination, for example: rice, nuts and greens.

Try to choose organic, animal produce and fish with scales – ocean-swimming or freshwater (not from fish farms) – rather than those with skins, and shellfish, which are scavengers and tend to live in the polluted estuaries and shallow waters. Eat any animal protein in small quantities only as excess can often contribute to constipation.

Buy nuts in their shells and dry-roast them at home. Commercial nut butters are often made with hydrogenated oil and easily become rancid. Look for unhydrogenated nut butters or, even better, make yor own.

Oils and fats

Cold-pressed oils (obtained from nuts and seeds) supply essential fatty acids which are vital to the health of the nervous system, skin, hormone production and the function of the immune system. They also reduce cholesterol levels.

They are best eaten raw, so use them in salad dressings, home-made mayonnaise or blend them with juice, yoghurt or food after cooking, as a natural supplement. A combination of olive oil with sunflower or safflower would make a balanced oil to use.

Hydrogenated fats and oils should be avoided, due to their toxic nature. (See *Cholesterol* on page 85.)

Use butter in moderation or use an unhydrogenated margarine for spreading and olive oil for cooking.

Fruit and vegetables

Fresh fruit and vegetables are an invaluable source of vitamins, minerals and trace elements. They also provide protein and fibre and should make up the bulk of the diet. Vitamin C (easily destroyed on exposure to heat, light or air) is of particular importance – boosting the body's immune system and promoting tissue healing. It also assists the absorption of iron by the body.

Their food content is affected by such things as long periods between picking and eating, cooking, transportation and artificial fertilisers. All this tends to cause a deficit of vitamins and minerals. So try to eat organically grown produce. Or, even better, try to eat home-grown.

Eat something raw before each meal, like a salad, a piece of fruit or vegetable. This helps to boost the immune system, plays down any immune reactions and tones the mucous membranes.

Water

Tap water can be contaminated with chemicals from agriculture or industry, phosphates, lead, aluminium, chlorine and fluoride, and hormones. All of these can be implicated in illness, especially allergies. Have your water analysed, then consider using a water filter which, depending on the water, will remove a proportion, if not the majority, of the contaminants. Mineral/spring waters vary in their contents, check the analysis.

Fluid intake is important to the body, which is largely composed of water, helping to flush toxins out of the system and maintaining fluid levels. 1 to 2 litres of water per day is the level required to replace fluids lost through breathing, sweating, passing urine and faeces, and for cleansing the system.

Salt

Salt is *hydrophilic*, meaning it loves water. In the body, too much salt can cause increased amounts of fluid held in the system, leading to increased blood pressure and water retention. Too much salt also leads to the loss of potassium and magnesium from the body in favour of sodium from the salt, and is implicated in arteriosclerosis.

Use a natural sea salt without anti-caking agents instead of standard table salt and limit the amount you use, perhaps gradually reducing the amount. Even better, use a herb salt and rely on herbs and spices to flavour your food.

Dairy products

Milk is specifically designed for the developing young. In the case of cow's milk, this is for the growing calf. Many people believe it is unnatural for adults to consume milk-products.

Milk is mucus-forming and should be avoided during colds and any catarrhal condition such as chest infections, sinusitis, and even thrush, to prevent further congestion in the body. Some conditions are a result of allergy to the protein in the milk. This is very common with asthma and eczema in children.

Like sugar, milk is present in a lot of foods – soups, cereals, processed foods, biscuits, as well as the more obvious cheese, yoghurt, ice-cream, custard and chocolate.

Alternatives to cow's milk include soya milk, yoghurt and ice-cream, almond or coconut milk, and sheep or goat products (although these can also cause sensitivity). Apple or grape juice instead of milk on cereal can be very palatable. Of all the dairy products, live yoghurt seems to be the best tolerated. Lack of calcium is often a concern, but nuts, seeds and green leafy vegetables are a rich, even superior source.

Alcohol

The consumption of alcohol easily becomes excessive in our society, with special occasions, social life and many work practices revolving around alcoholic drinks. A glass of wine or two with a meal is beneficial, but daily consumption in excess of this can cause health problems.

In excess, alcohol damages your liver and nervous system, and can affect your job and home life. Alcoholism is arguably the country's largest public health problem. The cost to the nation is immense, in lost working days from illness or hangovers, premature death, accidents, attacks on others and simple inefficiency.

Alcohol can contain a cocktail of chemicals, as it is only necessary to declare the strength of alcohol. So try to choose organic wines and additive-free beers.

Caffeine

Caffeine is a drug which acts as a stimulant to the nervous system, increasing adrenaline production, often making it difficult to relax. It interferes with hormone levels, and impedes the absorption of iron from the gut. The consumption of caffeine several times a day, day after day, puts considerable strain on the nervous system. Coffee, tea, chocolate, cocoa and cola drinks all contain caffeine.

Coffee is the major source, and even decaffeinated coffee still contains some caffeine. If you choose a decaffeinated coffee make sure the method used to extract the caffeine does not involve chemicals. Choose one that states it has been prepared via the Swiss water filter method.

Cutting down your coffee intake can cause headaches and make you feel generally unwell, as your body goes through the withdrawal effects of the caffeine. When you have a cup of coffee again, you might experience the shakes as the caffeine affects your nervous system.

Although nothing can replace the taste of real coffee, try changing to herbal teas, or coffee substitutes like Yannoh, Moccava, Bambu, Caro, Barleycup or dandelion coffee.

Fruit juices, drunk hot if preferred, or pure water are other alternatives.

Sugar

Sugar is a relatively new introduction into our diets, being an expensive luxury when it first came to this country. Today it is incorporated into so many food products it is difficult to avoid without reading labels carefully. It causes tooth decay, hypoglycaemia, can lead to late-onset diabetes, candidiasis and interferes with the function of the immune system. In children, sugar can cause hyperactivity, wakefulness, irritability and mood swings.

Sugar is used widely in commercial cereals, processed and tinned foods, cakes, biscuits, chocolate, ice-cream, jams and sweets.

White sugar is devoid of all nutrients, supplying only calories and robbing the body of vitamins and minerals.

Demerera sugar, in moderation, is better than refined white sugar, supplying some nutrients, with molasses providing a good source of vitamins and minerals.

Alternatives to sugar include real maple syrup, date syrup, organic honey (in moderation – it can still cause tooth decay) concentrated fruit juices like apple and pear, sugar-free jams made with concentrated juices, dried fruit and sweet, ripe fruit, like bananas and dates.

Wheat

Wheat tends to be part of our staple diet; it is also a common food allergen, perhaps due to introducing it to babies too early.

Coeliac disease is a severe intolerance to the gluten in wheat, rye, oats and barley, causing malabsorption, and usually diagnosed in children.

Wheat intolerance can also cause digestive and mental disturbances and since wheat is also a grass, it can aggravate the symptoms of hayfever.

It is worth checking the amount of wheat you are eating in a day, trying to restrict wheat to one meal a day.

Most people know that wholemeal products are supposed to be better for you but unless they are organic this means increasing your consumption of pesticides. Wholemeal uses the wholegrain, which includes the outside husk which contains the highest levels of pesticide residue. Indeed it may well be the pesticides rather than the wheat causing an allergy, so choose organic wholemeal flour, bread and pasta. Organic wheat also provides other important nutrients, like silica, which are vital for healthy bone structure.

The Hay diet

This diet is named after Dr Hay who instigated the principles of not mixing proteins and carbohydrates at the same meal. This means that carbohydrates like bread, potatoes and pasta should not be eaten at the same time as protein foods like meat, cheese and eggs because they need different acid-alkali conditions to be digested properly. This idea is quite foreign to the standard meat and potatoes but can be remarkably effective for digestive problems, allergies, arthritis and other complaints. The diet goes further into the mixing of alkaline and acid foods generally and the beneficial effects to health. For further information, read *Food combining for health* by Doris Grant and Jean Joice.

Supplements

Vitamin and mineral supplements are often regarded as necessary where modern farming methods have left food lacking in its supply of nutrients. However, multi-vitamin tablets tend to be synthetic in origin. It is better to choose organic foods, and if you wish, or need, to take a supplement, choose one which is naturally derived (see *Useful addresses* for suppliers). **Kelp, nettles** and **parsley** are examples of herbs which are good sources of vitamins and minerals.

Exercise and relaxation

Exercise boosts the immune function, aids the circulation of the blood and lymph, improves the elimination of waste products, enhances the sense of well-being and aids the ability to relax.

Relaxation is necessary to balance work and exercise. It is a time to recharge our batteries with vital energy so that we can appreciate life and function effectively in it. Ideally, relaxation should include quiet, reflective times, perhaps using meditation, but this is highly individual. Television and reading are probably the most common ways of relaxing in our society.

Breathing

Breathing is essential to life, bringing in vital oxygen and excreting the product of respiration, carbon dioxide. The lungs are also responsible for the excretion of other waste products and toxins – those produced by the body, the unwanted pollutants from the environment, or the mucus resulting from an infection or irritant to the lungs.

Correct breathing will help bring harmony and balance to your whole being.

Breathing techniques

Abdominal breathing is learning to breathe from your abdomen instead of your chest. Try abdominal breathing lying down in a relaxed atmosphere. If you put your hands gently on your abdomen you should be able to watch and feel the abdomen rise as you breathe in and fall as you breathe out. It can help to think of the breath in three stages – as it passes through the throat area, as it passes into your chest and makes your ribs expand, and then as it passes into the abdomen. Breathing out can be accentuated by pursing the lips and blowing gently. Hold your breath for a few seconds, the same length of time as the out breath.

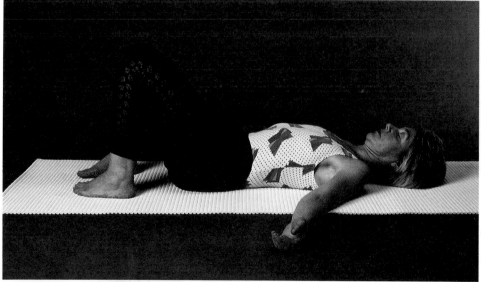

Yoga teaches relaxation and correct breathing

Gradually increase the duration of these breaths, and during normal activity check where you are breathing from, especially if you feel you are becoming tense. Going back to abdominal breathing can be most calming, and with practice gives control, and brings a sense of general well-being. To learn the discipline of breathing correctly, take up Yoga, T'ai chi or Chi Gung.

Smoking

On a physical level, smoking increases the heart rate and reduces the supply of oxygen to the blood. It also coats the lining of the lungs with tar and increases stomach acidity.

It can lead to bronchitis, heart disease and cancer. Apart from poisoning the system, it pollutes the atmosphere, subjecting non-smokers to passive smoking.

The herbs mentioned under *Stress* can help you give up the habit.

The role of herbs

Culinary herbs can be used every day to enhance health, as well as enhancing the flavour of the foods we eat. They can supply vitamins and minerals, protect from infection and promote digestion. **Parsley**, **garlic** and **cayenne** are typical examples of this dual function.

Herbs can be taken preventatively to support your body in times of stress and at the times of year when you are more susceptible to illness. For example, if you have a tendency to chest infections during the winter, **coltsfoot** can be taken, for up to three months to strengthen the lungs as winter approaches. If there are a lot of colds and 'flu around, **garlic** and **echinacea** can be taken to improve resistance.

Herbs can also be used to help clear the body of toxins that have built up in the body, supporting the liver in its difficult task in a polluted world.

When illness does occur, herbs can be used very effectively as the first line of treatment.

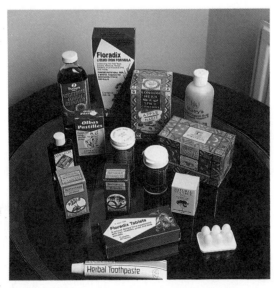

A selection of commercially available products

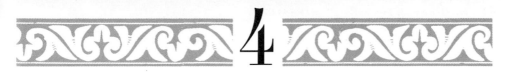

4

PREGNANCY AND CHILDBIRTH

Conception

A healthy pregnancy and baby require certain preliminaries in respect of diet and fitness, preferably prior to conception. However, this is not the woman's responsibility alone. It is important to look at the health and lifestyle of both partners, particularly if there are any problems in conceiving.

Consider any factors which are compromising your body, including alcohol consumption, smoking, caffeine intake, junk food, stress levels, working with VDU screens, and any health problems, past, present or hereditary.

It is best to leave at least three months between coming off the Pill and trying to conceive, as although it suits some women better than others, it usually leaves a degree of hormonal imbalance. This can be corrected using **agnus castus**.

The IUD or coil is associated with an increased risk of pelvic infection and ectopic pregnancy. Bear this in mind if you use this method of contraception or are thinking of doing so. Past use might have left a low-grade infection which could affect your chances of conceiving.

Infertility is permanent in only a small percentage of cases, so it is worth looking into any underlying factors before resorting to things such as fertility drugs and IVF.

Diet

Special attention to diet is required before and during pregnancy and breast-feeding. See the recommendations under *How to survive modern living* (page 25) and note the chemical build-up through the food chain.

Food can be a difficult subject in pregnancy, when intense likes and dislikes, alongside nausea and vomiting, disrupt the picture of ideal nutrition. However, a healthy diet and lifestyle prior to conception is certainly beneficial.

Most importantly, assess alcohol consumption and caffeine intake. Both affect the baby and can compromise the mother's health.

Protein is vital for the growth of the baby and needs to be sufficient for the mother's requirements too. This should consist of plenty of vegetable protein; animal products should ideally be organic.

Avoid eating refined carbohydrates (sugar, biscuits, etc.), junk food and additives.

Drugs and herbs during pregnancy

Orthodox drugs and any form of medication should, if possible, be avoided during pregnancy, particularly tranquillisers and aspirin. This is especially important in the first three months when the vital structures of the baby are being formed.

Herbs

If treatment is necessary, however, herbs can provide a safe, gentle alternative to orthodox drugs. Herbs are a balanced product whose constituents are easily assimilated by the body without any harmful side-effects.

Certain herbs should, however, be avoided during pregnancy, mainly due to their potential ability to contract the uterus. Some of these are employed during childbirth for this reason. Other herbs are more toxic by nature.

Herbs to avoid

Black cohosh	**Life root**
Barberry	**Mistletoe**
Blood root	**Mugwort**
Blue cohosh	**Pennyroyal**
Broom	**Poke root**
Cotton root bark	**Rue**
Feverfew	**Southernwood**
Golden seal	**Tansy**
Greater celandine	**Thuja (Arbor vitae)**
Juniper	**Wormwood**

- **Nutmeg**, **basil**, **cinnamon**, **rosemary**, **sage** and **parsley** should not be taken in large quantities.

- **Aniseed**, **caraway**, **celery, cumin**, **dill** and **fennel seeds** should also be restricted.

- Some essential oils should be avoided during pregnancy, as they are absorbed to a certain extent during massage. They are not for internal consumption unless prescribed by a qualified practitioner. These include: **aniseed, cinnamon bark, basil, bay, fennel, hyssop, juniper, marjoram, myrrh, nutmeg, oregano, pennyroyal, rosemary, savory, sage, thyme** but if you are in any doubt, ask a practitioner for advice.

Exercise, rest and relaxation

Fitness is ultimately important for stamina during the forthcoming labour. Exercise improves the circulatory system of the mother and thereby the oxygen available to the baby. It also assists the ability to rest, relax and breathe properly. Swimming, walking and yoga are all excellent during pregnancy.

Tiredness can be all-consuming in the first three months. The rise in progesterone levels relaxes the blood vessel walls, so lowering the blood pressure. To suggest rest seems laughable, if that's all you seem to be doing. Do not try to resist or worry about your need to rest.

The ability to relax is important. It pays to learn some breathing and relaxation exercises which you can use during labour. These are not complicated, and involve breathing so that your abdomen expands as you breathe in and contracts as you breathe out. Ante-natal or yoga classes can prove invaluable in helping you to practise the techniques.

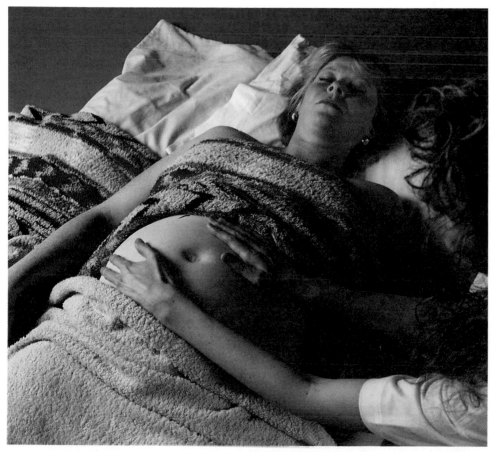

Massage with essential oils can help you relax and soothe away the general aches and pains of pregnancy

Smoking

It is preferable to review the smoking habits of **both** partners before
conception. Heavy smoking can cause toxicity that is harmful at the time
of conception and smoking during pregnancy (especially more than ten
cigarettes a day) affects the health of the placenta and the blood supply to
the uterus. The health of the baby is therefore compromised and labour
may be complicated by the generally decreased oxygen levels from a poor
blood supply. Women **and** men should give up smoking at least four
months prior to conception.

This information isn't encouraging if you are already pregnant and a
smoker. It is difficult to give up smoking and to do so can simply increase
tension levels. Seeking the help of a practitioner is advisable. See *Stress* in
An A–Z of ailments to deal with any tension associated with giving up
smoking.

Problems during pregnancy

Pregnancy can cause a variety of complaints, brought about through the
change in hormone levels, the need for organs like the kidneys and heart
to work much harder and the sheer weight and pressure of the baby as it
grows. These problems range from constipation and backache to
anaemia and high blood pressure. Refer to *An A–Z of ailments* for any of
these problems, but check the list of herbs to avoid, on page 34. It is also
advisable to check treatments with a medical herbalist, who might be able
to suggest something more appropriate to take during pregnancy.

Morning sickness

This can occur at any time of day and seems to be aggravated by tiredness
and low blood sugar levels. Whether you are suffering mild nausea or
severe vomiting, it can make life miserable. It is one of the first signs of
pregnancy, and tends to be accompanied by extreme tiredness and
lethargy. More often than not the problem stops at 12 to 14 weeks
gestation when hormone production is taken over by the placenta,
though it can continue throughout pregnancy.

The exact cause is unknown. The body is certainly going through
upheaval in these early weeks with a great surge of progesterone. The
drop in blood pressure, due to the relaxing effect of the circulating
progesterone, is no doubt contributary to the tiredness and lethargy
experienced. This can aggravate the nausea, particularly if associated
with a decreased blood supply to the brain – experienced if you feel dizzy
or faint on getting up.

It is certainly an effective way of making you rest during those
formative weeks and it is not detrimental to the baby.

Diet

Eat small, regular meals to keep your blood sugar levels stable, avoiding sugary, fatty and junk foods, and caffeine. This period of nausea and sickness is often accompanied by intense likes and dislikes of certain foods and smells. So if salads repulse you, just try to eat as well as you can.

- Try to have something to drink and eat before getting out of bed in the morning.
- When you go out, take a supply of dry biscuits with you to nibble as the need arises.
- Try eating some carbohydrate before going to bed, for example a piece of toast.
- Brewer's yeast and yeast extract can be helpful.
- Sparkling mineral water can bring effective relief of nausea.
- Try Sea Bands – these are wrist bands that work on acupuncture principles and are available from major chemists.

Exercise

Make sure you get enough fresh air and plenty of rest.

When to seek professional advice

If the vomiting is excessive and uncontrollable (*hyperemesis gravidarum*) dehydration can result which is potentially dangerous to the survival of the baby.

Herbs

- **Ginger** can be taken in tea form, using $\frac{1}{4}$ tsp per cup of the powder or a few slivers of fresh. Crystallised ginger root, ginger biscuits, ginger drinks, especially fizzy ones, can all be helpful (just watch the sugar content in these products). Gerard and Potter both make ginger tablets, and Arkocaps produce them as *Phytotravel*.
- **Chamomile**, **lemon balm** and **meadowsweet** are all soothing to the stomach. Make an infusion of 1 to 2 tsp per cup as required.
- **Peppermint** can be very soothing and also has a bitter action. Infuse 1 tsp per cup as required.
- **Gentian** has a more pronounced bitter action and is useful where there is a weak digestive system or poor liver function. It is best taken in tincture form. Take $\frac{1}{2}$ tsp in water 10 to 30 minutes before meals, or as required.
- **Black horehound** is a traditional remedy for morning sickness and is a relaxant to the digestive system. Infuse 1 to 2 tsp per cup, and have as required.

- **Slippery elm** or Spirulina could be taken as powder or tablets. Both are nutritious and soothing.

Pre-eclampsia

Characterised by high blood pressure, water retention and protein in the urine, pre-eclampsia is associated with toxaemia and can lead to eclampsia (convulsions). The onset is usually quite sudden. Signs include headache and seeing flashing lights. It is thought to be immunological and is most common with first babies. Pre-eclampsia is potentially dangerous to both mother and baby, and needs professional help. It is **important** to seek advice as soon as you suspect a problem. See *High blood pressure* and *Water retention* in the *A–Z of ailments*.

Diet

- Dietary changes can do much to help, and can prevent pre-eclampsia occurring.

- If you are showing symptoms, cut out all meat, alcohol and spices.

- Eat plenty of fruit and vegetables.

- Salt should be severely restricted.

- Rest is vital.

Stretch marks

Skin type plays its part in how prone you are to these. If the skin is not elastic enough to cope with expansion, stretch marks will appear. They can appear overnight on the areas of the body which expand rapidly during pregnancy – the abdomen, breasts and thighs.

Diet and supplements

- Eat plenty of cold-pressed oils to nourish the skin from the inside out (sunflower, safflower and olive).

- Pumpkin seeds are high in zinc, and sunflower seeds are high in zinc and silica (important in maintaining the integrity of the skin).

- Vitamin E is also important. A rich source is wheatgerm.

Herbs

- **Horsetail** is high in silica and can help build up tissue integrity. An infusion using 1 tsp per cup can be taken twice a day. Arkocaps' *Phytosilica* (bamboo) is an alternative.

- Massage the appropriate areas daily. Use avocado, **comfrey** (high in allantoin, remarkably healing), **marigold** or wheatgerm (high in vitamin E) oil as a base oil. Perhaps make a mixture and use almond, safflower or vitamin E oil to make a lighter massage oil.

- Essential oils of **lavender**, **mandarin** and **rose geranium** make a nice addition to the base oil. Dilute 1 drop of essential per 2 ml of base oil.

Preparation for childbirth

Hospital, home or domino (where your midwife comes into hospital with you for the delivery)? One of the most important aspects of the preparation is the environment in which you are planning to give birth. There is a choice open to you, so choose what is best for you. Informative books are listed at the back of the book and local NCT and home birth support groups can offer helpful advice.

If you are going to be attending your local hospital for the delivery, make yourself familiar with the environment and procedures of the place. Choice of room, furnishings (beds v. cushions, beanbags, stools), lighting, music, availability of a bathroom or birthing pool, can all play a part in your comfort and therefore in your ability to relax.

Choose the support of someone to be with you – your partner and/or a friend.

If you know who your midwife is going to be, you can get to know her and discuss your views about the birth. It is important that those around you during the labour know your wishes and respect them. You are unlikely to feel like arguing against intervention during delivery itself.

It isn't possible to plan the birth precisely, each one is different. However, being well-prepared, with an open mind to the possibility of compromise, will help.

Herbs

- **Raspberry leaf tea** can be taken after the third month to tone the uterus and prepare it for childbirth. Infuse 1 tsp per cup, and have 1 cup a day. This can be increased to 2 to 3 times a day after the sixth month. In a first pregnancy the uterus does not usually need as much toning as in subsequent pregnancies, so don't start taking it until the sixth month, when 1 cup a day will be sufficient. **Raspberry leaf** is also available in tablet form. Take half the suggested dose with a first pregnancy.

- **Squaw vine** is another traditional herb used for preparing the uterus for childbirth. It can be taken from the sixth month and should be taken for several weeks prior to the birth. Take as for **Raspberry leaf**.

Birth kit

It is worth organising some remedies that might be required during the birth process. A ready packaged kit can be supplied.

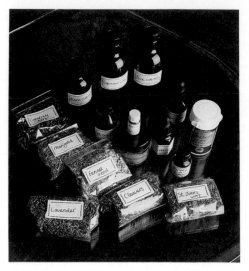

The herbal Birth Kit (available from the authors. See Useful Addresses)

Childbirth

This is a deeply personal affair, when time and space can come to mean nothing to you. Support rather than interference is more productive in aiding, what is after all, a bodily function.

Herbs

Many of the herbs contra-indicated during pregnancy come into their own during labour. They can help to stimulate and maintain regular contractions, while reducing the risk of post-partum haemorrhage.

- Herbs can be taken throughout labour, as drinks or sips of hot infusions or decoctions. Make these up in the usual way, using 1 tsp per cup, unless otherwise stated. They can be taken freely.

- Teas can be applied via compresses to the abdomen or back or added to baths.

- Drops of tincture can be taken under the tongue, or in a little water, 10 drops at a time, as often as every 15 minutes.

Induction

Black and **blue cohosh**, in equal parts, can be taken to tone the uterus and encourage contractions. If you have passed your due date, take a decoction of 1 tsp per cup twice a day. This might be easier to take in capsule form (2, twice a day), as it is quite bitter. Alternatively, take the tincture (5 ml twice a day).

Any of the herbs mentioned for weak contractions below can be used in a mixture.

Acupuncture, cranial osteopathy or reflexology might also be employed.

Pain management

This can be a major preoccupation and cause a good deal of anxiety during pregnancy. It is difficult to anticipate how painful labour will be, especially if this is your first baby. Pain threshold levels vary from one person to the next so it is worth keeping your options open. The biggest key to coping with pain, and maintaining control, is by being comfortable in the environment in which you are giving birth, and having the support of someone close to you.

- Controlled deep-breathing through your contractions can be very effective in dealing with the pain. This doesn't involve complicated techniques, but practising abdominal breathing helps (see *The art of breathing* by Frederick Leboyer).

- Ante-natal classes, yoga and relaxation tapes during pregnancy are all good preparation. Tapes with music and relaxations can be played during the labour.

- Firm massage to the lower back helps to relieve pain and discomfort.

- A foot massage can be comforting and restorative.

- Use essential oils of **chamomile**, **clary sage** and **lavender** in a massage, 10 to 20 drops in 10 ml of base oil. These are relaxing and help to deal with the pain. You might be very sensitive to perfumes, so choose your favourite oils. They can also be used in an oil burner in the room.

- Water has a remarkable effect on reducing pain and irritability. If you are interested in using a birthing pool look into the availability of one at your hospital. They can also be hired for home use. You don't have to have a special pool to benefit from water – a bath or shower can bring relief. Add essential oils and herbs to the water, as required.

- **Yellow jasmine** is a painkiller and sedative available under a prescription from a qualified herbalist.

- A TENS machine is an alternative to drugs, available in most hospitals (and can be hired privately). Broadly speaking it works on acupuncture principles. Many women find it useful in early labour, though it can become irritating and can't be used in conjunction with water.

- Entonox (gas and air) is the least intrusive form of drug relief, though not to every woman's liking. It is usually only needed towards the end of labour, if something additional to the above methods of pain relief is needed.

- Pethidine and epidurals are more invasive and will affect your ability to control the labour, so more intervention is likely. Pethidine can adversely affect the baby, making it floppy at birth.

Contractions

- If your contractions are weak and irregular, labour doesn't really get going, but is nonetheless tiring. A mixture of equal parts of **black** and **blue cohosh** as a decoction or tincture will help to encourage regular contractions.

- If the labour is long, and tiredness is affecting the strength of the contractions, **feverfew** or **mugwort** can be taken as an infusion or tincture.

- **Golden seal** is an excellent stimulant and tonic to the uterus. Make a decoction with ½ tsp per cup, and just take drops if it is too strong to sip. Alternatively, use the tincture.

- **Clove**, **myrrh** and **rosemary essential oils** will help stimulate contractions and boost energy levels. Use 10 to 20 drops in 10 ml of base oil (any vegetable oil will do). This can be massaged into the abdomen and lower back.

- An infusion of **cloves** (6 to 12 per cup) and **rosemary** could be sipped as a tea. 1 drop of **myrrh oil** may be added to this. This mixture could also be applied as a compress or added to a birth pool or bath.

- Contractions might be very strong, frequent and painful, but last an ineffectual amount of time. Relaxants are needed to deal with the general tension and any feelings of fear. **Chamomile**, **lavender**, **limeflowers**, **motherwort**, **skullcap** or **valerian** could be used.

- **Black** and **blue cohosh** can be used to regulate the contractions, with a decoction or tincture of **cramp bark** acting as an antispasmodic to the uterus.

- Essential oils can be used in a massage, or an oil burner to calm and soothe. See under *Pain management* for appropriate oils.

- Take **ginseng** as drops of tincture under the tongue to boost your energy and drink **raspberry leaf tea** with honey, adding Potter's *Composition Essence* or a pinch of **cayenne**.

Perineal rigidity

The herbs mentioned above for strong contractions will generally help to deal with tension in this area.

Hot compresses can be applied directly to the perineum. You might add **cramp bark** (a decoction of 2 tsp per cup), or **lobelia**, which is obtainable under prescription from a qualified herbalist. They are both antispasmodic.

Delivery of the placenta

When the placenta peels away from the uterine wall it leaves an open wound, so it is important to prevent excessive blood loss. It is also important to ensure that none of the afterbirth tissue is retained, as this can lead to infection.

Breast-feeding helps, as it causes the release of oxytocin which stimulates the uterus to contract and expel the placenta. Any of the herbs used for weak contractions will also promote the expulsion of the placenta.

Beth root, **periwinkle** and **shepherd's purse** will stimulate uterine contraction and also astringe the blood loss, thereby allaying the risk of post-partum haemorrhage.

Caesarean section

If you know you are going to have a Caesarean delivery, you have time to prepare yourself and decide whether you will have an epidural or general anaesthetic. Homoeopathic **arnica** taken before and after the operation will reduce bruising.

If the operation is an emergency, take homoeopathic **arnica** and **Bach flower rescue remedy** to deal with bruising, shock and trauma. The herbs suggested under *Perineum*, on page 44, can be used to promote speedy recovery and minimise scarring.

Post-natal care

For your new baby

Add **chamomile** and **lavender** as an infusion or a few drops of oil to the bath water to help to soothe the baby. This is especially indicated if the labour was traumatic, but every baby needs to adjust to his/her new world.

Rescue remedy could be used if the labour was difficult, or very quick, or if the baby was born by Caesarean.

The cord usually heals well by itself and antibiotic applications are counter-productive to the natural process. Should there be any infection, or the cord is slow to heal, **calendula** cream or ointment with **tea tree oil** can be applied.

Lavender tea can be used to wash the cord.

For you

Herbs can be used to heal and restore your body after childbirth.
Raspberry leaf will help your uterus to contract efficiently, thereby

reducing any risk of haemorrhage. It will induce your milk flow and balance your hormones after the birth.

Perineum

Damage to this area will depend on the amount of bruising caused through pushing, if you have torn, or if you have had an episiotomy.

Pelvic floor exercises as soon as possible after the birth will improve the circulation to the area and start to build up tone.

It is important to avoid becoming constipated as this will create pressure on the perineum. Have plenty of fibre in your diet and brave the first urge to pass a stool.

Use ice-cubes to reduce swelling or cold applications of the herbs below.

Herbs

- **Comfrey leaf**, **marigold**, **lavender** and **St John's wort** can be made up as an infusion to add to a bidet or equivalent. Use 1 oz (25 g) in 1 pint (500 ml) of boiling water. Increase this proportionally if adding it to the bath. You can add more boiling water to the herbs for a second brew.

- Leaving out the **lavender**, the above mixture can be taken as a tea, 2 tsp per cup twice a day.

- **Arnica**, taken homoeopathically, will help with bruising and soreness, as will **distilled witch hazel** (chilled perhaps) which can be applied to the perineum.

- **Lavender** and **myrrh** can be added to a bath or bidet in the form of essential oils. These promote healing and help prevent infection.

- **Arnica** (**not** applied where the skin is broken), **calendula** or **comfrey** ointment could be used, as could **St John's wort** oil.

- If you have had an episiotomy, **comfrey** and **St John's wort** are useful to use in massaging the scar tissue.

- Wheatgerm oil with a few drops of **lavender essential oil** could also be used as a massage.

- Sea salt in the bath water can bring relief and stave off infection. If you have had stitches, check that this won't dissolve them before time.

Depression

'Baby blues' are common sometime within the first few days. This is when the milk starts to come in and many women feel tearful. The hormones change dramatically after the birth and need time to settle down. There may, of course, be more fundamental issues to be dealt with. If this is the case, it is important to share your feelings with someone. Depression combined with tiredness makes it difficult to cope, making your baby vulnerable to your moods.

Try to have rest and some time to yourself and ask for help if you need it. Make sure you are eating properly and include cold-pressed oils such as sunflower or safflower in your diet. Brewer's yeast will provide necessary B vitamins.

Herbs

- **Borage**, **lemon balm**, **oats**, **St John's wort** and **vervain** are all restorative and can be taken as a mixture or singly. Have an infusion of 2 tsp per cup 2 to 3 times a day.

- Hormone normalisers such as **agnus-castus** and **raspberry leaf** can prove beneficial. They need to be taken over a period of at least three months.

- **Agnus-castus** should be taken as an infusion first thing in the morning only, using 1 tsp per cup. Gerard do *Agnacast* tablet.

Uterus

After-pains can be quite severe, particuarly after subsequent births. They are caused by the contractions as the uterus reduces in size and may be more noticeable when breast-feeding. **Black haw** or **cramp bark** are antispasmodic to the uterus. **Black** and **blue cohosh** can also be used.

Blood loss, or *post-partum haemorrhage*, is usually alleviated if homoeopathic **arnica** and the herbs mentioned under *Weak contractions* and *Delivery of the placenta* have been taken during labour. Floradix iron formula is excellent to re-build reserves, especially if you have lost a lot of blood.

Although it is normal to bleed for up to six weeks after giving birth it is important to contact your midwife if you have a dramatic loss of blood.

The oxytocin released during breast-feeding causes the uterus to contract, thereby speeding up involution (the uterus returning to its normal size). **Raspberry leaf** tea or **squaw vine** will aid the process.

Breast-feeding

Breast milk is best for your baby. It helps to protect against infection, is nutritionally superior and easier for your baby to digest than bottle-feeds. It is also an ideal medium for administering herbs to your baby!

Engorgement

This tends to happen when the milk first comes in and when there is a long interval between feeds.

To relieve the discomfort and get the milk flow going, bathe the breasts in warm water or apply warm flannels. This will soften the breasts sufficiently for the baby to be able to latch on and feed properly.

Alternatively, the milk can be expressed and frozen for future use.

Mastitis

Mastitis can develop if a duct becomes blocked when the breasts become engorged. An ill-fitting bra or any pressure on the breast can also cause a blocked duct. At the first sign of inflammation (watch for any red patches on the breast) or tenderness it is important to act. Untreated it can rapidly lead to a temperature and 'flu-like symptoms.

Massage the area with a stroking action from the fingertips, moving towards the nipple.

Cabbage leaves inside the bra can help.

Encourage regular feeds, or express the milk.

Herbs

- **Calendula** can be taken as a tea (infuse 1 to 2 tsp per cup 2 to 3 times a day), or applied to the breast via compresses, poultices or cream. It is anti-inflammatory, anti-infective and specific for the lymphatic system.

- **Cleavers** is also specific for clearing the lymph tissue. Have an infusion of 2 tsp per cup 3 times a day.

- **Echinacea** should be taken as an anti-infective. Gerard do this in tablet form, as do Arkocaps as *Phytokold*.

- **Lavender**, as well as helping with the infection, is soothing. It can be taken as a tea or applied externally.

- **Dandelion root** may be used. Make a decoction of 1 tsp per cup twice a day.

- **Fresh ginger root**, peeled and made into a decoction using the equivalent of 1 oz (25 g) per pint (500 ml), can be applied as a compress to the breast. It stimulates the circulation and has antiseptic properties.

- **Poke root** can be very effective but should be prescribed by a qualified herbalist.

- **Distilled witch hazel** will soothe and quell the inflammation. Apply as often as required.

Milk flow

Make sure that you are drinking plenty of fluids. This is important in maintaining your milk supply.

Adequate nutrition is vital as the demands being put on your body's resources are enormous. You might find your appetite increases with breast-feeding, even if it's already good. Don't restrict your food intake – you are more likely to lose weight than gain it!

Rest might seem impossible to achieve when you are having to meet the demands of your new baby but try to rest when your baby sleeps. Enlist help from family or friends, especially if you have other children at home. The first month is an important time to recuperate after the birth, physically and emotionally, so don't over-extend yourself.

Floradix iron formula is good insurance against becoming depleted and helps to re-build energy levels after the birth.

Herbs

The herbs which stimulate milk flow are called *galactogogues*.

* **Borage** and **vervain** act as tonics to the nervous system, as well as stimulating milk flow.

* **Agnus-castus** increases prolactin secretion (responsible for stimulating milk production) and is a hormone balancer.

* **Fennel**, **aniseed**, **dill** and **caraway seeds** are galactogogues and carminatives. They are especially useful if your baby has colic as they are administered through the breast milk.

* **Nettles** and **raspberry leaves** are very nutritious and enrich the milk.

* Other useful herbs are **goat's rue**, **marshmallow leaf** and **milkthistle**.

* All the above can be made up as infusions. If using seeds, crush them first in a pestle and mortar, or with a rolling pin. Use 1 tsp per cup 2 to 3 times a day.

Too much milk

This is not usually a problem when breast-feeding.

The engorgement experienced when the milk first comes in settles down as it adjusts to your baby's requirements.

If you cannot breast feed, or when you want to stop **red sage tea** will help to reduce the milk flow. Infuse 1 tsp per cup 2 to 3 times a day.

Sore and cracked nipples

This can be a problem particularly with a first baby when the nipples haven't toughened up yet. It is fundamental to make sure your baby is latched on properly when feeding (seek the advice of your midwife or NCT breast-feeding counsellor).

Expose your breasts to the air as much as possible, avoid wearing a bra at night and let the nipples dry naturally after feeding. You can rub some breast milk over the nipple at the end of a feed. Honey can also be applied. A nipple shield can be used if the situation becomes desperate.

Herbs

* **Distilled witch hazel** is soothing and can be applied to the nipples as often as necessary.

* **Calendula** ointment will speed healing.

5

CHILDREN

It is important to respond quickly to the first signs of illness in a child before waiting to see what happens. Most childhood illnesses are self-limiting but it is still better to act preventatively through diet and herbs and by making sure your child has enough rest.

Whooping cough, for example, is virtually impossible to diagnose until the whoop starts, when treatment is difficult. Boosting your child's immune system (see page 12), removing dairy products from the diet, not letting the child get over-excited or over-tired and treating the cold and cough as they manifest, can do much to lessen the severity of the illness and prevent complications.

Most parents know when something is not quite right with their child. Initial signs of illness include poor appetite, sleeping more, restlessness, irritability, lethargy, crying for no apparent reason, or any change from normal behaviour. Always consult a practitioner if your child develops a rash or skin eruption, as it may indicate the start of a notifiable illness.

Using herbs with children

Seeing a sick child can be as distressing for the parent as the illness is for the child. The wish to alleviate the suffering as quickly as possible is normal. However, the administration of powerful drugs, such as antibiotics, steroids, sedatives or painkillers, can have life-long repercussions. (Antibiotics destroy the body's normal, protective ecology of bacteria; steroids interfere with the healing process by suppressing inflammation; strong sedatives and painkillers dull the vitality and ability of the child to function fully.) There is a place for these drugs – one wouldn't question the use of antibiotics in meningitis, for example, but too often they are handed out as if they are the only answer. Children respond remarkably well to herbal medication. More often than not, a gentle herbal remedy will be more effective than a powerful drug and will not have unwanted side-effects.

We should regard childhood illnesses as stages in our children's development. A fever should be viewed as the normal response of a healthy body. It is Nature's way of ridding the body of toxins and should not be impeded by administering drugs to suppress the temperature unless it goes above 39°C (103°F). It is of course important to keep a careful eye on the progress of a fever, especially in young children where temperature regulation is still not fully developed. Much can be done herbally and with water to check a fever without impinging on its positive effects.

Herbal medicine is wonderfully versatile and does not have to be the concoction of foul-tasting remedies often imagined. Herbs can be administered as poultices, linaments, hand- and footbaths, via the bath, as ear- or nosedrops, ointments, capsules or tablets, drops, syrups and teas that are soothing and pleasant to take. See *The natural pharmacy* on page 16.

Vaccination

Viewing disease as a positive part of childhood brings up the vexed question of vaccination. Whether to vaccinate your child or not is an extremely difficult decision to make. Vaccination does not guarantee that your child will not get the disease and there is evidence connecting vaccination to long term auto-immune diseases like arthritis. Moreover, recently vaccinated children can infect other children. It is worth considering the alternatives, particularly where there is an allergic tendency in the child or the family.

However, if you are thinking about not vaccinating your child, it is important to equip yourself with as much information as you can, and to discuss the issue with different practitioners.

Diet during childhood

Appetite

Children's appetites vary greatly from one child to another. They can vary from day to day, with fads for certain foods coming and going. Your child might eat bananas every day for several weeks, then not touch another one for a month.

Children have a strong sense of what they need and fulfil their nutritional requirements by eating appropriately. It is self-defeating to attempt to force children to eat what they don't like, but do keep introducing new foods for them to try.

Weaning

Careful weaning can be critical for a child's immune system and future development and if there is any history of allergy in the family special care needs to be taken.

The majority of commercially produced baby foods and drinks contain unnecessary sugar which taints the baby's palate for the future. They can also cause hypersensitivity, making your child irritable, fractious, hyperactive or have sleep problems. See page 29 for alternatives to sugar.

Dairy products, wheat, eggs and oranges, are among the most common allergenic foods. Too early exposure to these can set up a sensitivity to them. Do not introduce these into your baby's diet until he or she is 10–12 months old, especially if there is an allergic history in the family. Again, many commercial baby foods contain these foods, so it is important to read the labels carefully.

The best foods to give in the first year are vegetables, fruit, rice, ground nuts and seeds. Meat is unnecessary when children are very young and might be difficult to digest and constipating.

When first introducing solid foods, give only one food at a time, so that if there is a reaction you know what is causing it. Sensitivity to a food can cause colic, diarrhoea, irritability, catarrh or a skin rash. If there is a reaction, wait at least a month before introducing it again. The best foods to introduce initially are puréed carrot, pear or apple. Leave any foods that you or your partner are sensitive to till last, along with wheat etc. Introduce no more than one new food a week.

Choose a time for meals when your child is not over excited or too tired to eat. Make sure they are having enough fluid when going on to solids. Be relaxed and don't worry about the mess when self-feeding starts!

Diet during infections

During any acute illness, keep children on a light diet. Most children lose their appetite anyway. Don't force them to eat as it will only put more strain on their system.

If there is a fever, just give plenty of fluids – pure water, herb teas, diluted fruit juices.

Don't give any dairy produce, sugar or meat, especially with catarrhal conditions of the respiratory tract or stomach.

When the acute stage is over, serve plenty of fruit and vegetables and soups rich in vegetable protein. Beetroot juice can be given diluted with water, carrot or apple juice to boost the immune system.

Valuable supplements include Floradix and natural vitamin C.

Administering herbs

Apart from the usual teas and tinctures which can be made into syrups, sweetened with honey or disguised with liquorice, herbs can be effectively administered via baths, poultices and eardrops. See *The natural pharmacy* on page 16.

Suppositories are a very effective and under used method of administering herbs. They are especially useful for children who find it difficult to take medicine or where giving herbs by mouth is not always possible, for example, during an asthma attack. As the herbs bypass the digestive system, they are directly absorbed into the bloodstream, so effecting a speedy treatment.

Dosages for children

Standard doses and how to combine the herbs into mixtures is outlined on page 21. Generally speaking, halve the dose for children and quarter the dose for babies. Children over 12 can be given $\frac{2}{3}$ of the standard adult dose, or even the full dose, depending on their body weight.

For example, when preparing an infusion for a baby, use $\frac{1}{4}$ tsp of herb per cup. If this is going to be mixed with juice or diluted with water, use only a $\frac{1}{4}$ of a cup of water to infuse the herb and then add the juice or water.

For tinctures, use 5 to 10 drops for babies up to 2 years old. If you are breast-feeding you can administer the medication via your breast milk, in which case take a standard adult dose. From 2 to 5 years old use 20 to 40 drops, and from 5 to 12 years $\frac{1}{2}$ tsp of tincture.

These doses are to be taken 2 to 3 times a day, except during times of acute illness, like a fever when the dose can be taken every 3 hours.

Another way to work out the dosage for a child is to take their age next birthday and divide it by 24, so a child of 8 takes $\frac{1}{3}$ of the adult dose.

When using essential oils with children, the above also applies. Make sure you dilute essential oils in a bath dispersant or base oil before adding to the bath. Use 2 to 3 drops of essential oil with babies, and 5 drops per bath from 2 years old. When making up an oil to apply, to the chest for example, use 1 drop of essential oil in 5 ml of base oil for babies and 1 drop in $2\frac{1}{2}$ ml for children over 2 years old.

Herbs suitable for children

It is important to bear in mind that only the mildest herbs are necessary for treating children. Those to have on hand in the house should include: **catmint**, **chamomile**, **boneset**, **echinacea**, **elderflowers**, **hyssop**, **limeflowers** and **thyme**.

It is useful to have some **liquorice**, as small amounts help to disguise and sweeten strong-tasting mixtures. It is also soothing for coughs and a mild laxative, so helping to keep the bowels moving during an illness.

The essential oils and ointments suggested for a basic dispensary on page 22 should also be on hand.

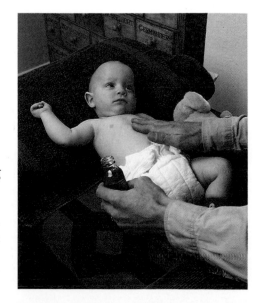

An A–Z of children's illnesses

Adenoids (enlarged)

The adenoids are part of the immune system. They come up when the body is fighting an infection or there is some allergic reaction. When inflamed, they interfere with breathing, make the speech sound nasal and can interfere with hearing. See *Tonsilitis* and *Ear infections*.

When to seek professional advice

If it is a recurring problem.

Diet and supplements

- See *Diet during infections* on page 50.

Herbs

- **Cleavers** is a wonderful lymphatic tonic. Take 1 tsp per cup 3 times a day.

- **Echinacea** tablets will boost the immunity, as will beetroot juice, which most children like if mixed with apple or grape juice and diluted with water.

Chickenpox

This is a contagious, viral illness which spreads via droplet infection (talking, coughing, sneezing) and through contact with pustular spots.

It chiefly affects children under ten and can be caught from someone with shingles, as it is a related virus.

The incubation period is 14–21 days. It is most contagious just before the spots appear and until all the blisters have dried up.

First symptoms include headache, fever and malaise. The lymph glands might be swollen. The spots appear on the trunk first, then the face and limbs. The scalp, the inside of the mouth and throat, ears, soles of the feet and anus or vagina can be affected.

The spots turn into oval-shaped, fluid-filled blisters within 24-hours and dry up in a few days. They can be very itchy and every effort should be made to encourage your child not to scratch them, to prevent scarring and setting up any skin infection. The spots come in crops, every 3–4 days, so there are spots present in different stages at the same time. All the spots should dry up and the scabs fall off in 10 days. Complications are rare but include encephalitis, pneumonia and kidney disease. See *Fevers*.

When to seek professional advice

- If spots develop on the eyeball.
- If your child is on steroids or immunocompromised in any way.
- If your child feels unwell or there is vomiting, headache or malaise after the spots have healed.

Diet and supplements

- See *Diet during infections* on page 50.

Herbs

- Take **echinacea** every 3 hours.
- Dab the irritating spots with distilled **witch hazel** (ideally cold) to take the itching away and prevent them becoming infected. A drop of **peppermint oil** can be added to 1 ml of **witch hazel** to make it more cooling.
- **Myrrh**, **golden seal** and **marigold** tinctures can be used as a lotion.
- Externally, **lavender**, **chamomile** and **tea tree oil** can be added to a lotion.
- **Galium** and **burdock** can be used during the eruptive period, internally and externally. **Poke root** is very effective but needs to be prescribed by a qualified herbalist.
- Use **St John's wort oil**, **comfrey**, **calendula** and **lavender** cream to counteract scarring.
- Poultices of **marigold** and **sage** will greatly ease any throat discomfort.

Colic

Many babies suffer from colic, most commonly in the first three months of life and usually at its worst in the evening and during the night.

Colic can be due to the baby not being correctly attached on to the nipple or feeding too quickly, so swallowing a lot of air with the milk.

With bottle-fed babies, it can be due to an allergy to the milk formula or air from the bottle.

Diet and supplements

- If you are breast feeding, keep off the foods that you went off during pregnancy.
- Stay off onions, garlic, beans, cabbage, soya products, and spicy foods, as these often upset a baby's tummy.
- Go on to the Hay diet yourself if breast-feeding, see page 30.

Herbs

- **Fennel** and **dill seed** are *carminitive*, which means they reduce intestinal wind.
- **Chamomile** poultices placed on the tummy or diluted **chamomile oil** rubbed into the abdomen soothe any muscle spasm.
- Gripe water works well. It is readily available from chemists and is now alcohol-free.

Ear infections

Babies and young children are particularly prone to ear infections due to their short eustachian tube, which easily becomes blocked when tonsils or glands are swollen or there is catarrh.

Due to risk of infection spreading to the bony parts of the ears and brain, treatment needs to be prompt.

Antibiotics are not the answer, especially when given repeatedly for persistent ear infections. They can drive the infection deeper as they don't resolve the underlying problem, even if they appear to work quickly. See *Adenoids (enlarged)*, and *Catarrh* and *Earache* in *An A–Z of ailments*.

Fevers

Fever is Nature's way of helping to beat off infection, so it must not be suppressed. However, if the temperature goes above 39°C (103°F), intervention is essential, and it is advisable to consult your doctor or a medical herbalist. Sponging or bathing your child with tepid water will help to lower and stabilize the temperature.

Diet and supplements

- See *Diet during infections* on page 50.

Herbs

- Give **echinacea** every 3 hours during the acute period.

- **Eucalyptus** and **thyme oil** rubbed on the chest and back will act as a strong antibiotic. It works especially well on chest infections but is always worth employing in fevers. Use 1 to 2 drops of essential oil per 5 to 10 ml of vegetable oil.

- **Boneset**, **limeflowers** and **elderflowers** are the best herbs to give during a fever.

- **Catmint** can be given to help reduce a fever. Give every hour, if necessary.

German measles (Rubella)

Spread by droplet infection, the incubation period is 2 to 3 weeks. Although mild in children, it tends to affect older children, adolescents and young adults more severely.

If it develops during the first four months of pregnancy, it can cause congenital malformation, such as heart or mental defects, deafness or cataracts.

The disease is not usually suspected until the rash appears as small, flat, pink spots behind the ears and on the forehead and then spreads rapidly to the trunk and then the limbs.

If the rash is dense, the skin looks red.

Mild conjunctivitis (red eyes) is common.

Tender enlargement of the neck glands usually occurs.

The illness lasts 2 to 3 days at most.

Herbs

- Give **echinacea**, **chamomile**, **burdock**, **boneset** and **lavender** internally.

- Use distilled **witch hazel** externally to reduce the irritation of the rash.

Glandular fever

The virus that causes glandular fever can debilitate people for years. It usually strikes in the late teens, around exam or other stressful times but can occur in children too.

'Flu like symptoms occur during the first part of the illness, followed by debility, inability to concentrate and, possibly, personality changes. Tiredness, malaise, headache, fever, swollen glands in the neck, a sore throat (with red spots), and a rash are all early symptoms. See *Fevers*, *Tonsilitis*, and *Convalescence* (page 13).

When to seek professional advice

- It is wise to have help from the beginning, in order to lessen the extent of the illness.

Diet and supplements

- The main item to put into the diet is beetroot as juice, raw or cooked root.
- Just give liquids during the fever, then plenty of fresh foods, especially fruit and vegetables.
- Spirulina and Floradix and vitamin C are beneficial supplements.

Herbs

- Give **marigold**, **wild indigo**, **echinacea**. Make a mix of these with **cleavers**, **dandelion root**, **nettles** and **vervain** and give 3 times a day for as long a time as it takes your child to become completely well.
- It is essential that you give **cleavers** in order to properly restore the lymphatic system.
- **Poke root** needs to be prescribed by a medical herbalist.
- **Eucalyptus**, **lavender**, **pine**, **rosemary** and **thyme** oils can be added to the bath water or rubbed over the chest and back during the acute period.

Hyperactivity

Overactive, uncontrollable children can be exhausting. It is hard to remember that their behaviour is not their fault but is caused by an irritation to the nervous system that keeps provoking them into activity.

Try to remove the irritant and then soothe, calm and heal the nervous system. See *Sleeplessness*, and *Allergies* in *An A–Z of ailments*.

Diet and supplements

- Remove sugar-containing foods.
- Remove all chemicals, whether stabilisers, anti-caking agents, preservatives, colourings or whatever.
- Remove tea, coffee, chocolate, cola drinks and cocoa, as all contain caffeine and are therefore stimulating.

Herbs

- **Limeflowers**, **vervain**, **chamomile** and **lemon balm** are all calming, soothing and healing to the nervous system. Make tea with any one or a mix.

- **Hops** can be added to the bath or placed in a pillow. For the bath, put a small handful in a muslin bag, under the hot tap.

Measles

Measles is a highly contagious, viral illness common in childhood.

The incubation period is 8–14 days. It is spread by droplet infection – talking, coughing and sneezing, and is infectious from 7 days after infection to 10 days after the rash started.

It starts similarly to a cold, with nasal catarrh, sneezing, red, watering eyes, swollen eyelids, and headache.

A cough and hoarseness, due to laryngitis, and photophobia (sensitivity to light) come by the second day.

Koplik's spots, white spots surrounded by a red area of inflammation inside the cheeks or around the parotid duct, are diagnostic of measles.

During the third or fourth day of the highly infectious catarrhal stage, the rash starts behind the ears and hairline and rapidly appears over the rest of body, accompanied by a high temperature. These flat, brownish-red spots fuse to form the characteristic blotchy rash which usually covers the face but does not itch.

The rash is fully erupted in 2–3 days and the fever subsides as the rash disappears.

Swollen lymph nodes in the neck, vomiting and diarrhoea, abdominal pain and earache can occur.

Complications include middle-ear infection and pneumonia due to secondary infection. Persistent conjunctivitis can lead to corneal damage if unattended. Most cases are uncomplicated but stomatitis, gastroenteritis, appendicitis and encephalitis can result. Immunized children may only get respiratory symptoms but they are still infectious. See also *Fevers*, and *Conjunctivitis* in *An A–Z of ailments*.

When to seek professional advice

- If your child isn't feeling better after a week.

- If the temperature starts to rise again.

Diet and supplements

- See *Diet during infections* on page 50.

Herbs

- Give **echinacea** as tablets, as tea or added to the bath to ease the discomfort.

- Give **thyme**, **burdock** and **chamomile** as tea 3 to 4 times a day.
- Add 10 drops of **eucalyptus** or **lavender oil** to the bath.
- Bathe eyes, if sore, with cool **elderflower** or **chamomile** tea.

Mumps

This viral illness, spread by droplet infection, usually affects school children and young adults.

The incubation period is 18 days. Fever, malaise and spasms of the jaw muscles is followed by swelling of one or both of the parotid glands (at the angle of the jaw), which may in fact be the first symptom. The submandibular glands (under the jaw) may also be swollen. The symptoms subside in a few days and may be followed by the swelling of the previously unaffected gland.

When to seek professional advice

- If abdominal or testicular pain occurs.
- If a severe headache or stiff neck develops.

Diet and supplements

- See *Diet during infections* on page 50.

Herbs

- Give **cleavers** and **marigold** tea to aid the lymphatic tissue.
- **Echinacea** will also help, as tablets or tea every 3 hours, or added to the bath water, 1 tbs brewed in 1 pt boiling water and poured in.

Nappy rash

Nappy rash is caused by the interaction of urine and faeces. It can be made worse by some foods, such as oranges, making the faeces or urine stronger.

Disposable nappies have adhesives and other chemicals that react with the urine and can cause nappy rash in sensitive children.

Washable nappies should not be washed in biological washing powders and need to be rinsed thoroughly.

Children with allergies or skin conditions and cradlecap tend to be more prone to nappy rash and the rash is often worse during teething.

Herbs

- Protect the bottom from irritating substances by using beeswax-based **calendula** cream at night and allowing air over the area during the day.

- **St John's wort oil** with **lavender essential oil** is excellent.

Sleeplessness

Children need to sleep at least 15 hours a day as newborn, gradually reducing to about 8 hours as a 12 year-old (with some variation, obviously). If they are not having anything like this then there must be something keeping them awake.

Certain foods can irritate the system preventing restful sleep. Chemicals such as additives, colourings, preservatives, foaming agents or those present in the environment can also cause sleeplessness.

When to seek professional advice

- If the situation is intractable, seek help – sleep deprivation is unhealthy for you and your child.

- If your child is obviously in pain.

Diet and supplements

- Avoid tea, coffee, chocolate, cola drinks, foods with **any** additive.

- Sugar, honey and other sweet foods make children more energetic. This energy has to be burnt off, making children uncontrollable and unable to sleep.

Herbs

- **Chamomile** can work beautifully. Use it as tea in the bottle for babies and toddlers and as normal tea for older children.

- Put essential oil of **chamomile** in the bath, 5 drops per bath.

- **Limeflowers** can also prove helpful.

- Try some **hops** in the bath.

Teething

Teething seems to be accompanied by all sorts of other problems, such as nappy rash, diarrhoea, spots, colds and ear problems due to the stress put on the immune system by the pain and inflammation in the gums.

Herbs

- Rub 1 to 2 drops of **chamomile essential oil** on to the gum, no more than twice a day.

- Give a fractious child **chamomile** as tea.

- Woodwards do a *Teething Gel* that contains **gum myrrh**, **sage** and bee propolis and is widely available.

Tonsilitis

Inflamed tonsils occur when infection is being fought off or there is a chronic allergic response from the immune system. The tonsils are lymphatic tissue and need support to carry out their protective function, rather than being removed unnecessarily. See *Adenoids (enlarged)*

When to seek professional advice

- If the condition is recurrent.

Diet and supplements

- See *Diet during infections* on page 50.

Herbs

- A gargle will ease the situation, if the child is old enough. See *Sore throat* in *An A–Z of ailments* for details and alternatives.

- Give **cleavers tea** to restore the lymphatic tissue.

- **Echinacea** will also help, either as tablets or as tea, 1 tsp per cup 3 times a day.

Whooping cough

This is a contagious, childhood illness caused by a bacteria which occurs most commonly in the under 5s.

The incubation period is 7–14 days until the catarrhal stage. This stage is highly infectious and is accompanied by a runny nose, conjunctivitis and an unproductive cough. It is almost impossible to diagnose during this very contagious stage. After about a week, however, there are severe coughing bouts (the paroxysmal stage), usually at night, which end in the characteristic whoop, and perhaps vomiting.

The paroxysmal stage can last a couple of weeks, with symptoms gradually declining over the subsequent weeks but the cough can persist much longer.

It is the very young who are most at risk, especially the newborn, whose air passages are narrow and lungs immature. Congestion and coughing can seriously diminish the oxygen supply to the brain, causing convulsions. There can be serious consequences but usually only if your child's health has been compromised previously by environmental or hereditory factors.

Vaccination does not mean your child will not get whooping cough.

When to seek professional advice

Whooping cough is a notifiable disease so contact your doctor as well as a qualified herbalist.

Diet and supplements

- See *Diet during infections* on page 50.

Herbs

- See *Coughs* and *Bronchitis* in *An A–Z of ailments* for advice on employing herbs to relieve the spasm, dealing with the infection and using inhalations and vaporisers to keep the atmosphere moist.

- If whooping cough is in your area, or your child has been in contact with an infected child, give precautionary measures, such as **hyssop** and **coltsfoot** tea, every day.

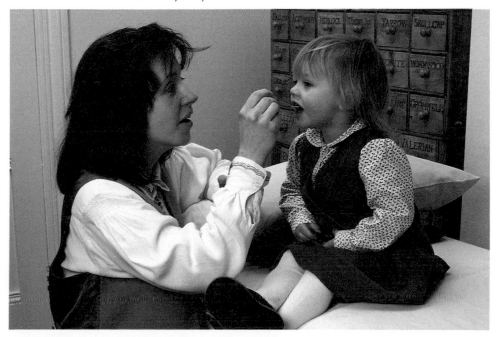

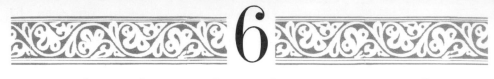

6

AN A–Z OF AILMENTS

Abscesses

These are accumulations of pus which can occur anywhere in or on the body. Commonly due to a focus of infection, they are a sign of congestion and toxicity. When acute, they become inflamed and painful, often accompanied by a raised temperature, as the body attempts to fight the infection.

When to seek professional help

Recurrent abscesses indicate the need for thorough investigation to rule out any chronic disease, such as tuberculosis. Whatever the cause, they require professional attention. This might involve draining the abscess and should always be accompanied by a cleansing regime through diet and herbs. See *Boils*.

Acne

Acne is generally associated with adolescents, where it reflects the changing hormone levels and emotional difficulties of becoming an adult. However, this condition can also appear later in life.

It occurs when the skin's sebaceous(oil) glands become blocked. These then become infected, causing spots that can leave disfiguring scars. The face, chest and back are the areas most usually affected.

Poor elimination, for example constipation, and a bad diet need to be corrected.

If the condition persists after adolescence, or, if you are a woman and it is worse premenstrually, it could be aggravated by a hormone imbalance.

The condition can also result from steroid treatment or pituitary or hypothalamus disease.

Assess any chemicals that are being used or drugs that are being taken.

Cleanliness is important but avoid using harsh chemicals that dry the skin. See also *Constipation*, *Premenstrual tension*.

When to seek professional help

If the condition does not show signs of improvement after a couple of months of consistent treatment, see a qualified herbalist to find out what is causing the acne.

Exercise

- This is important to improve the circulation of blood and lymph, so aiding the elimination of toxins.

- Fresh air and sunlight are also beneficial in skin problems.

Diet and supplements

- Dairy produce should be limited to plain, live yoghurt.

- Caffeine, soft drinks, sweets and junk food should be avoided, as should fried and fatty foods.

- Include in your diet some raw, cold-pressed oils.

- **Evening primrose oil** capsules could be taken as a supplement.

- Brewer's yeast, pumpkin seeds and wholegrains are rich in zinc which aids the healing process.

- Try to drink 1 to 2 litres of pure water a day.

- See *What is a healthy diet?* on page 25.

Herbs

- **Echinacea root** is antiseptic and stimulates the immune system. Have a decoction of 1 to 2 tsp per cup 3 times a day.

- **Cleavers tea** is essential to clear the lymphatic tissue. Take an infusion of 1 to 2 tsp per cup 3 times a day.

- **Dandelion root** stimulates the liver, which is the detoxifying organ of the body. Take this as a decoction of 1 to 2 tsp per cup 2 to 3 times a day, or roast, grind and prepare like filter coffee.

- **Nettles** are nutritious and cleansing and can be taken as an infusion of 1 to 2 tsp per cup 3 times a day.

- **Blue flag** stimulates the lymph, circulation and bowel and **burdock** is an effective tissue cleanser. These can be made up as a decoction using $\frac{1}{2}$ tsp of the root per cup and taken 2 to 3 times a day. Ideally, add some warming herb to your brew, such as a few grains of **cayenne** or the tip of a teaspoon of **ginger** to each cup.

- **Chamomile**, **lavender** and **marigold**, made up as an infusion of 2 tsp per cup, can be used to wash the face. These herbs are anti-inflammatory, anti-infective and healing. Alternatively, use this mixture in a facial steam bath to open up the pores and help draw out some of the impurities. Distilled **witch hazel** makes an excellent toner to use afterwards. It can be used at any time to cleanse and soothe and it is anti-inflammatory.

- **Comfrey** cream can be used as a healing agent to counteract the scarring.

- **Calendula** (marigold) cream is also healing.

- **Lavender**, **myrrh** and **tea tree** essential oils are all antiseptic. Add 10 drops to a facial steam bath or add to the **comfrey** or **calendula** cream, using 1 drop of essential oil per 10 ml of cream.

- If the condition is hormone-related, **agnus-castus** is a hormone balancer which acts on the pituitary gland. Infuse ½ to 1 tsp of the crushed berries per cup, to be taken in the morning. This need only be taken for the second half of the menstrual cycle in women, until the period starts.

- Men can also take **agnus-castus**, but something like **saw palmetto** or **damiana** might be more appropriate.

Available products

Arkocaps' *Phytoderma* (burdock), *Phytokold* (echinacea).
Gerard's *Echinacea* or *Echinacea and Garlic* tablets, *Blue Flag Root Compound* tablets (also burdock, sarsaparilla). *Agnacast* tablets (agnus-castus) can be taken as a hormone balancer.
Potter's *Skin Clear* tablets (echinacea), *Elixir of Echinacea* (also fumitory, wild indigo), *Alterative Tablet No. 34* (red clover, sarsaparilla, queen's delight, blue flag, burdock).
Weleda's *Ankedoron Lotion* and *Deep Cleanser*. Weleda also makes a good range of skin products based on herbs and oils.

Allergies

These are caused when the body's immune system reacts to internal or external substances that are not necessarily harmful to the body. The liver, which is the detoxifying organ of the body, becomes taxed with the amount of chemicals it has to process. When the liver becomes overburdened, there is a tendency for the defences of the immune system to become sensitised to everyday substances. Drugs further compound the problem, putting added strain on the liver. When the defences fight against the body's own tissues, the reaction is termed as *auto-immune* (see page 13).

Food allergies can often be traced back to the introduction of dairy produce or wheat at too early an age. It is advisable not to introduce the most allergenic foods – wheat, milk and milk products, eggs, sugar and oranges – until a baby is at least ten months old, twelve months if there is a family history of allergy-related problems.

Breast-feeding helps to boost a baby's immune system and reduce the risk of allergy. However, although breast is still best for your baby, chemicals and sensitivity to certain food substances can be passed to the baby through the breast milk.

The reliance on a relatively small group of foods, such as bread, milk, cheese and eggs which are eaten every day, also contributes to the incidence of food intolerance.

Allergies can present in many ways – as skin reactions, for example eczema and urticaria; as respiratory problems like asthma, catarrh and hayfever; as digestive symptoms such as diarrhoea, constipation and stomach pain; as well as headaches, migraines, high blood pressure, tiredness, hyperactivity and insomnia. See also *Asthma, Eczema, Hayfever, Liver disorders, Stress.*

When to seek professional help

Due to the complex nature of allergies it is advisable to work in conjunction with a practitioner, especially when embarking on a restricted diet.

Diet and supplements

- Eat organic foods and cut out all junk and processed foods, additives, caffeine, sugar and any suspected foods. See *What is a healthy diet?* on page 25.

- Try a day of fasting (see page 12) once a week or once a month.

- Balance the amount of any one food you have.

- The Hay diet (see page 30) can be very helpful.

- Aim to eat a varied diet, with different grains, pulses, nuts, seeds and fruits and plenty of vegetables and include cold-pressed oils in the diet.

- **Evening primrose oil** can be taken as a supplement.

- Take $\frac{1}{2}$ to 1 tablespoon of apple cider vinegar diluted in warm water with a little honey to taste first thing in the morning, and up to 3 times a day. This helps to boost the immune system and detoxify the body.

Herbs

- Take **dandelion root** to support and cleanse the liver.

- Take **burdock** to cleanse the tissues and **celery seeds** and **nettles** to flush toxins out of the body.

- Take **borage** and **liquorice** to support the adrenal glands.

Anaemia

Whatever the cause, anaemia results in the blood being less able to supply oxygen to the tissues. Diagnosis is by measuring the amount of haemoglobin in the blood.

Symptoms include breathlessness, lethargy, palpitations.

It is important to discover the reason for the anaemia, so consult a qualified practitioner. Causes include pernicious anaemia, and a deficiency in vitamin B12, folic acid or iron. This deficiency may be dietary, or an inability to absorb the essential nutrients for making healthy red blood cells from the digestive system.

Excessive menstrual bleeding will use up iron reserves, leading to anaemia, as will any continued blood loss, for example from a stomach ulcer.

There is also a relative drop in haemoglobin levels during pregnancy, due to the production of red blood cells not quite keeping up with the increasing blood volume.

When to seek professional help

If you suspect you may be anaemic ask your practitioner for a blood test. It is important to find out the cause of the anaemia, and to rule out pernicious anaemia or any other blood disorder.

Diet and supplements

- Ordinary tea (and caffeine in general) will inhibit the absorption of iron, especially when consumed with a meal. Bran (from wholegrains) and legumes (peas, beans and pulses) will also inhibit iron absorption. So you may need to assess and reduce your consumption of these.

- To build up your iron reserves, eat plenty of the following: apricots, beetroot, black cherries, green leafy vegetables (especially raw), molasses, watercress and parsley.

- Vitamin C improves the absorption of iron. It is interesting to note that fruit and vegetables high in iron also contain vitamin C.

- Free-range eggs are a particularly well-balanced protein food and contain iron, vitamin B12 and folic acid.

- A traditional source of dietary iron, liver, should be from organically raised animals only.

- A glass of red wine with a meal will improve absorption and supply iron at the same time.

- Swedish bitters or Angostura bitters, available from your off-licence, can be used to promote digestion and absorption.

- Brewer's yeast and spirulina are good nutritional sources of iron and B vitamins. Floradix iron formula is an excellent supplement if you are anaemic.

- Iron tablets can cause constipation and imbalances in the body, especially if the anaemia is not due to iron deficiency. Natural sources of iron are much easier for the body to assimilate and do not cause constipation.

Herbs

- **Dandelion leaf**, **nettles** and **raspberry leaf** provide iron. Make an infusion using 1 to 2 tsp per cup of one or all of them and take once or twice a day.

- **Dandelion leaves** can be added to salads and the young tips of **nettles** make a delicious, spinach-like soup!

- **Yellow dock** and **burdock** are high in iron. Grind the root of either and put it into capsules. Take 2 capsules a day. Alternatively, obtain the tincture and take $\frac{1}{2}$ tsp of this twice a day before meals.

- **Gentian root** will improve the digestion and absorption of iron. It is very bitter and is therefore best taken as a tincture, $\frac{1}{2}$ tsp 2 to 3 times a day before meals.

Available products

Potter's *Infusion Gentian Compound Concentrated.*

Angina (pectoris)

This is chest pain caused by lack of oxygen to the heart muscle, due to an insufficient blood supply. Narrowing of the arteries that supply the muscle might be due to hereditary narrow blood vessels, furring up and hardening of the arteries, or general tension and anxiety.

Taking stock of life and assessing work and leisure activities can do much to avert the serious consequences associated with angina.

Smoking impairs the circulation and supply of oxygen to the tissues so should be stopped. See *Anxiety, Arteriosclerosis, Cholesterol, Circulatory problems* and *Stress*.

When to seek professional help

It is advisable to seek the guidance of a medical herbalist, especially if you are taking any drugs for the condition.

Diet and supplements

See under *Arteriosclerosis* and *Cholesterol* for appropriate dietary advice.

Exercise

- Gentle exercise, increased gradually, is vital. Check with your practitioner to establish the level of exercise you should start with.

- Relaxation and breathing exercises are also of great benefit, as they help to release tension from the heart and allow better blood flow.

- Yoga and T'ai chi would be most appropriate disciplines to learn and practise.

Herbs

- **Hawthorn berries** nourish and help to strengthen the heart, and **cramp bark** is antispasmodic to the muscle walls of the arteries. Make a decoction of this mixture, 1 tsp per cup and take 3 times a day.

- **Hawthorn flowers**, **lime flowers** and **lemon balm** are all relaxing and have an affinity to the heart and circulation. Make an infusion of equal parts, using 1 to 2 tsp per cup and have this tea 3 times a day.

Available products

Gerard's *Hawthorn* and *Cramp Bark* tablets.

Anorexia and bulimia

Anorexia nervosa is a complete aversion to food, leading ultimately to starvation. It is associated with extreme weight loss and absence of menstrual periods in women.

Bulimia nervosa exists where any food consumed is deliberately vomited up. It is associated with food binges following a sense of heightened appetite.

Both can involve the abuse of laxatives and other weight control drugs.

This obsession with weight is most commonly associated with adolescent women and is potentially life-threatening if left untreated. See also *Anxiety*, *Depression* and *Stress*.

When to seek professional help

If anorexia or bulimia is suspected, it is vital to seek help. Counselling is imperative, and vitamin and mineral supplements are best taken with the advice of a qualified practitioner.

Exercise

- Massage, especially aromatherapy, can help with accepting your body.

- Breathing and relaxation exercises, yoga and T'ai chi can all prove beneficial, especially in the long-term.

Diet and supplements

- Zinc deficiency is a common cause of the problem and can be easily tested for by tasting a zinc solution (ask your practitioner or a chemist about this). If someone is zinc deficient, there will be no taste, if not, it will taste repellent. A zinc deficiency can come about through dieting and eating junk food. This mineral is required in increased amounts with the start of puberty.

- When the condition is under control, careful attention to diet and perseverence are required to help the digestive system function fully again.

- Drink fruit and vegetable juices if you are not eating solids yet.

- Wholegrains, nuts and seeds will be too difficult for the digestion to cope with initially.

- Start with soups and steamed or mashed vegetables.

- White grapes are an easily digested and nourishing food.

- Porridge is an excellent convalescent food and is restorative to the nervous system.

- Chicory and endive are bitter vegetables which help to stimulate the appetite and digestive juices.

- Artichokes, globe or Jerusalem, help the liver and digestion.

- Consider the Hay diet (see page 30) to aid digestion.

- Coffee, tea, chocolate, cocoa and cola drinks should be avoided, as the caffeine they contain will simply stress the under-nourished nervous system.

- Raw cold-pressed oils like sunflower, safflower and olive, and brewer's yeast which is high in the B vitamins, are important to build up the nervous system.

- **Evening primrose** with/or **borage oil** should be taken.

- Floradix liquid iron formula and liquid herbal supplement supply essential nutrients.

- Spirulina is an algae which is highly nutritious and contains the B vitamins. This is available as powder or tablets.

- Swedish bitters or Angostura bitters, which are available from your off-licence, can be taken, ideally 10 to 30 minutes before eating, to stimulate the appetite and digestive system.

Herbs

- **Dandelion root** can be taken as a decoction, using 1 tsp per cup 2 to 3 times a day before meals, or roast and grind the root and make up like filter coffee. This is a bitter tonic to the liver and digestive system.

- **Gentian root** is particularly effective. It is a digestive stimulant, and it is also anti-inflammatory. Make a decoction using $\frac{1}{4}$ tsp per cup to have 2 to 3 times a day before meals. It is, however, very bitter and might be easier to take as tincture, $\frac{1}{2}$ tsp before meals. Bitters stimulate the appetite and promote the digestion. Their work begins when they come into contact with the taste buds, so the liquid form is preferable to tablets or capsules.

- **Centaury** aids a debilitated digestive system. **Vervain** is a tonic and restorative to the digestive and nervous systems. **Agrimony** is healing to the digestive tract and will help with any acidity. Any of these herbs can be made up as an infusion using 1 tsp per cup to have 2 to 3 times a day.

- **Chamomile**, as well as being calming, is anti-inflammatory and soothing to the digestive tract. Have an infusion of 1 to 2 tsp per cup 2 to 3 times a day.

- **Slippery elm** as powder or capsules will help with any pain from acidity. It will protect the digestive tract (in bulimia the constant vomiting is very destructive to the mucous membranes), and is also nutritious.

- **Liquorice** is anti-inflammatory and protective to the digestive tract. It is also a support to the adrenal glands which become depleted when the body is stressed with such a long-term illness. The natural root can be chewed, or a decoction made using $\frac{1}{2}$ to 1 tsp of the root per cup. Take this 2 to 3 times a day.

Available products

Gerard's *Papaya Plus* tablets (slippery elm, hydrastis, charcoal, papain) contain an active enzyme to help digestion.
Potter's *Appetiser Mixture* (chamomile, calumba, gentian), *Infusion of Calumba Concentrated*, *Infusion of Gentian Compound Concentrated*.

Anxiety

Most people suffer from anxiety at some time during their lives. A certain amount of worry is only natural, especially at certain times, such as before an exam or job interview, but if it becomes constant, it is getting out of control and needs treatment. See *Depression, Stress*.

When to seek professional help

- If the anxiety is taking over your life and is not being resolved.
- If you are becoming dependent upon drugs (or herbs) to control the anxiety.

Exercise

- Breathing and relaxation techniques help to bring control and peace.
- Yoga or T'ai chi are excellent activities to take up but any form of exercise that is enjoyable to you is beneficial.
- Baths or massage with some relaxing, essential oils can help enormously.

Diet and supplements

Cut out tea, coffee, chocolate, cocoa and cola drinks, as the caffeine in these is stimulating the nervous system where the reverse is required. Replace these with herb teas, such as *Golden Slumbers* (London Herb & Spice Company) and *Sleepytime* (Celestial Seasonings) which can be drunk during the day as well as before going to bed.

Herbs

- **Chamomile** and **lime flowers** are relaxing and soothing. **Lavender** and **lemon balm** are calming and uplifting. **Skullcap** and **vervain** act as tonics as well as relaxants to the nervous system. **Passionflower** and **valerian** are traditional and more specific sedatives to counteract tension and poor sleep. Have an infusion of 1 to 2 tsp per cup of your chosen herb/s 2 to 3 times a day. However, **valerian root** is particularly pungent and might be more acceptable in capsule form.
- Essential oils such as **chamomile**, **clary sage**, **geranium**, **jasmine**, **lavender**, **lemon balm**, **marjoram**, **patchouli** and **rose** could be used in the bath or in a massage oil. For a massage, use 10 drops of essential oil per 20 ml of base oil (a vegetable oil such as grapeseed is ideal). For a bath, add a total of 10 drops to the water. Coconut oil could be used to disperse the essential oil.

Available products

Arkocaps' *Phytocarm* (passion flower) and *Phytotranq* (valerian).
Gerard's *99 Tablets* (hops, passiflora, valerian), *Motherwort Compound* tablets (also passiflora, limeflowers), *Biophylin* tablets (valerian, skullcap, Jamaican dogwood, black cohosh).
Potter's *Newrelax* (hops, skullcap, valerian, vervain) or *Passiflora* tablets.
Cornucopia, Neal's Yard and Weleda all do excellent relaxing bath products.

Arteriosclerosis

Commonly known as *hardening of the arteries*, arteriosclerosis involves degeneration of the artery walls. Fat deposits fur up the arteries causing thickening and loss of elasticity of the vessel walls. Calcification of the arteries is common in long-standing degeneration. The passage of blood through these vessels is made difficult, so the perfusion of oxygen to the tissues slows down. It is associated with high blood pressure, diabetes, high cholesterol levels and smoking. It can affect any of the arteries in the body, including the ones that supply the brain.

Attention to diet, exercise, and stopping smoking can lead to a significant improvement in the condition. See also *Angina, Cholesterol* and *Circulatory problems*.

When to seek professional help

Arteriosclerosis is a progressive condition which can vary in severity. It might be part of a wider problem, such as diabetes, or associated with taking orthodox drugs to reduce high blood pressure or to thin the blood. Seek a medical herbalist for advice.

Exercise

Gradually increase daily exercise. Walking, swimming and yoga are examples of activities that will help. Check with your practitioner the level of exercise acceptable for you to start at.

Diet and supplements

- See *Cholesterol* for appropriate dietary advice on fats and reducing blood cholesterol levels.

- Consumption of sugar is particularly detrimental. Products containing sugar abound, not just cakes, biscuits and chocolate, but cereals, tinned and processed foods and drinks.

- Salt intake also needs to be curtailed. It is probably easiest to achieve this by gradually reducing the amount you use. Herb salt or a salt substitute such as *Ruthmol*, composed of potassium chloride (if you have a kidney disorder, check with your practitioner about using this) can replace ordinary salt.

- Avoid salty cheese (like cheddar), yeast extracts (which have an extremely high salt content), foods in brine, salted nuts and convenience foods.

- Include spicy foods like **cayenne**, **ginger** and **horseradish** in your diet as they help to stimulate the blood flow.

- **Garlic** should be eaten daily and can be included in salad dressings or added to cooking. If the thought of eating fresh garlic worries you, take **garlic capsules** which are widely available from health food shops and chemists.

Herbs

- **Cramp bark** helps to dilate the arteries due to its relaxing effect on the muscular artery walls. Have a decoction of 1 tsp per cup 2 to 3 times a day.

- **Lime flowers** have a reputation of guarding against arteriosclerosis and healing the blood vessel walls. They are also relaxing and help to lower high blood pressure, especially where this is due to anxiety and tension. Have an infusion of 1 to 2 tsp per cup 2 to 3 times a day.

- **Ginkgo** is another valuable plant, which works particularly well where there is insufficient blood flow to the brain. It helps to open up the arteries and can reduce dizziness and poor memory. **Rosemary** also stimulates the circulation, particularly to the head and is associated with improving the memory. Both these herbs can be taken as an infusion of 1 to 2 tsp per cup 2 to 3 times a day.

Available products

Arkocaps' *Phytomemo* (ginkgo).
Gerard's *Cramp Bark*, and *Ginkgo* tablets.

Asthma

Asthma is a sudden and acute attack of difficult breathing, caused by spasmodic constriction of the airways. It is characterised by a wheezy chest and difficulty with breathing out. The accumulation of mucus in the airways, as a result of inflammation or infection, compounds the problem.

The cause is multifactoral with allergic, hereditary and emotional factors all playing a part. Viral and bacterial infections cause a significant proportion of asthmatic attacks. House dust and mites, feathers (for example, duvets and pillows), animals, smoke, household sprays and cleaning fluids, perfumes, exhaust fumes and other pollutants, moulds, grasses, pollen, can all trigger an attack.

The long-term use of steroids and inhalers exacerbates the problem. See *Allergies, Anxiety, Bronchitis, Catarrh, Hay fever, Stress.*

When to seek professional help

Asthma is a potentially serious condition, and is best dealt with in conjunction with a practitioner, especially if the asthma is being controlled by orthodox drugs (steroids and inhalers), and you wish to reduce your use of these. There may also be associated heart problems which need to be assessed.

Exercise

- Deep breathing exercises are very beneficial (see page 31).
- Gentle exercise, like walking or swimming, will improve your lung capacity.
- Consider taking up a wind instrument to improve your breathing.

Diet and supplements

- Generally improving the diet can help matters. See *What is a healthy diet?*, page 25.
- Dairy products are the commonest cause of sensitivity and create a lot of mucus. Eggs, bananas, oranges, wheat and peanuts can also cause sensitivity.
- Avoid sugar and refined carbohydrates, coffee, tea, chocolate and other caffeine-containing products which constrict the airways.
- Avoid all food additives and colourings, especially sulphur dioxide (E220), commonly used as a preservative in dried fruits and wine.
- Include plenty of **garlic**, onions and leeks in your diet.

Herbs

- **Thyme** is antispasmodic, antiseptic and an expectorant, so helps to dilate the airways and deal with the mucus and any infection. **Eucalyptus** is antiseptic and checks the excessive secretion of mucus in the airways. **Hyssop** is a relaxing expectorant and antispasmodic. Any or all of these can be taken as an infusion of 1 to 2 tsp per cup 2 to 3 times a day.

- Strong infusions of the above herbs could also be used in the bath, or as a compress applied to the chest during an attack.

- **Ephedra**, **lobelia** and **thornapple** are stronger herbs, which might be indicated but can only be prescribed by a qualified herbalist.

- Essential oils of **eucalyptus**, **hyssop** and **thyme** can be used externally to relieve spasm and congestion. Use 4 drops of **eucalyptus** and **thyme** to 2 drops of **hyssop**.

- For a chest rub, dilute 10 drops of the essential oil in 20 ml of vegetable oil and apply to the chest and back. Ten drops can be added to a bowl of hot water for a steam inhalation or added to the bath.

- If there is a lot of wheeziness at night, use 10 drops of essential oil in a vaporiser, or use an oil burner and keep the atmosphere moist.

- Ten drops of essential oil can be added to 1 pint (500 ml) of hot water to make a hot compress to apply to the chest.

- Olbas oil is a widely available decongestant.

- **Caution:** If your asthma is of a very allergic nature, proceed cautiously with the use of essential oils, as they might trigger a sensitivity.

Available products

Arkocaps' *Phytocoff* (thyme), *Phytoseptik* (eucalyptus).

Athlete's foot

This is a fungal infection that affects warm, moist feet. See *Candidiasis*.

Action

Bathe your feet daily and dry thoroughly. Wear cotton socks and leather or canvas shoes. Change your shoes so that you do not wear the same ones day after day.

Diet and supplements

- Athlete's foot thrives on a sugary diet, so cut out all sugar. This includes sugar in proprietary cereals, tinned and convenience foods, cakes and biscuits.

- Alcohol (fermented sugar and starch) also needs to be strictly avoided.

- Include **garlic**, leeks and onions in your diet.

Herbs

- **Marigold flowers** can be used to soak the feet in as they are antifungal and healing. Make an infusion with a handful of the flowers per pint (500 ml). Brew twice for extra strength.

- **Tea tree essential oil** is a strong, antifungal agent, so add 1 tsp to the marigold footbath.

- **Calendula** (marigold) cream with 10 drops of **tea tree essential oil** per 10 ml of cream, or 10 drops of **tea tree essential oil** in 10 ml of cold-pressed olive oil (which also has antifungal properties) can be applied to the feet after bathing.

- **Garlic oil** (see page 19) can be applied to the feet.

- **Lavender** and **thyme** might also be used, either as the infused herb or as an essential oil.

Available products

Mistry and Weleda both make a calendula talc.

Backache

Backache is largely caused by misalignments and muscle spasm. It can, however, be due to referred pain from an internal organ, perhaps a kidney infection or stomach ulcer, or there may be disease of the bone itself. Stress is also a factor in a large number of back problems. See *Osteoarthritis*, *Osteoporosis*, *Rheumatism and Arthritis* and *Stress*.

When to seek professional help

- A visit to an osteopath or chiropractor is advisable to assess and treat any misalignment in the spine.

- Massage can help to deal with muscle spasm and general tension.

- If you have persistent low backache that is perhaps associated with urinary symptoms, it is important to rule out any kidney involvement.

Exercise

Swimming and yoga can help to strengthen the back and relieve discomfort. Exercise is important and will help, especially where tension is an underlying factor.

Diet and supplements

Organic wholemeal bread, lettuce, raw spinach, parsnips, tomatoes and sunflower seeds are good providers of silica, which is vital to the health of the connective tissue.

Herbs

- **Horsetail** is high in silica and strengthens the ligaments of the spine. Have an infusion of 1 tsp per cup twice a day. It is also a tonic to the urinary system.

- Where there is a history of kidney weakness, an infusion of **parsley piert** can be taken, 1 to 2 tsp per cup twice a day.

- **Horsechestnut** is indicated where there is disc involvement and any accumulation of fluid causing nerve pressure. Have an infusion of 1 tsp per cup, or ½ tsp of the tincture twice a day.

- **Cramp bark** is beneficial where there is muscle spasm, along with **valerian**, which is a relaxant. Make a decoction using 2 tsp per cup and apply as a compress. Tincture can be used instead and applied with cotton wool.

- **Lobelia** is an excellent antispasmodic herb, available under prescription from a qualified herbalist.

Available products

Arkocaps' *Phytosilica* (bamboo).

Bad breath (halitosis)

Dental hygiene is obviously important but bad breath can commonly be attributed to a digestive problem or constipation. See *Constipation, Gum disease, Indigestion*.

Diet and supplements

- The Hay diet (see page 30) will aid proper digestion.
- Avoid dairy products and fried and fatty foods.
- Eat plenty of fruit and fresh vegetables, especially raw, at the start of each meal.
- Artichokes, chicory and endive stimulate the liver and digestive system, while fresh **mint** and **parsley** clear the palate.

Herbs

- **Peppermint** tea, 1 to 2 tsp per cup, as needed, can be used as a mouthwash to freshen the breath. It can also be drunk to help digestion.

- **Dandelion root**, 1 tsp per cup, or **gentian root**, ½ tsp per cup, as a decoction, half an hour before meals will stimulate the digestive system, as will Angostura bitters, available from your off-licence. Take ½ tsp in water 10 to 30 minutes before meals.

Bilious attack

The pain, nausea and headache associated with this digestive complaint are caused by the inappropriate secretion of bile from the gallbladder. It can be triggered by a fatty meal and may be due to the formation of gallstones.

The tendency towards gallstones is increased with taking the contraceptive pill or steroids, or being overweight.

Gallstones can get stuck in the neck of the gallbladder or the bile duct causing biliary colic. If the bile duct is blocked, it will produce jaundice. Inflammation or infection of the gallbladder usually accompanies gallstones. See *Cholesterol, Indigestion, Liver disorders*.

When to seek professional help

If you have gallstones, treatment is best undertaken with a medical herbalist, and unless you are accustomed to fasting, this should be supervised by your practitioner. Inflammation of the gallbladder commonly needs hospitalisation.

Diet and supplements

- If you can, give the gallbladder a rest for two weeks by eating only fresh fruit and raw vegetables. Drink 2 litres of apple juice a day and use the juice of 2 lemons and 4 tablespoons of olive oil on a salad each day. This will help to cleanse the gallbladder and allow any small gallstones to pass. After the two weeks are up, maintain a diet that contains plenty of fruit, especially apples, grapes and grapefruit, and vegetables.

- Avoid meat, margarine and anything fried or fatty.

- Dairy products can be eaten in moderation, especially live, plain yoghurt.

- Include apple juice, olive oil and lemon juice in your daily diet. Combined with plenty of dietary fibre, this will keep the gallbladder functioning fully and protect against the formation of gallstones.

Herbs

- **Fumitory** will ease the spasms of the gallbladder. Use 2 tsp per cup and drink freely.

- **Dandelion root**, 1 to 2 tsp per cup as a decoction, will stimulate the gallbladder. A decoction of **barberry** or **golden seal**, using ½ tsp per cup, could also be used. Continue taking the herbs for two weeks.

- Strong **chamomile** and/or **peppermint** tea (2 tsp per cup) can be enough to ease the discomfort.

- **Marshmallow** herb will soothe the inflammation of the gallbladder and gall duct and ease the passage of gallstones.

Available products

Arkocaps' *Phytodigest* (artichoke).
Potter's *Black root* and *Euonymus* tablets (also kava, burdock), *Infusion Gentian Compound Concentrated* (flavoured with bitter orange and lemon peel).

Boils

These are localised infections of the hair follicles and tend to occur when you are debilitated or after an over-indulgent diet.

They are an attempt by the body to clear toxins out of the system. The normal routes of elimination may be choked or not functioning fully. Sluggish circulation of blood and lymph, poor diet, and over-prescription of antibiotics may be causative factors. See *Abscesses*, *Circulatory problems*, *Constipation*.

When to seek professional help

Frequent boils can be due to an underlying problem, for example diabetes, so obviously need to be investigated.

Exercise

Plenty of exercise is necessary to increase blood and lymph flow, so that toxins can be mobilised and eliminated from the body.

Diet and supplements

- Beetroot is an excellent immune stimulant, as is **garlic** which is an antiseptic.

- Apricots, **parsley**, watercress and raw spinach are rich in iron and vitamin C and help to build the blood.

- Restrict your intake of dairy products to live, natural yoghurt.

- Avoid refined carbohydrates, especially sugar, cakes and biscuits.

- Avoid coffee, tea, chocolate, cocoa and cola drinks.

- Drink, if possible, 1 to 2 litres of pure water a day. See *What is a healthy diet?* on page 25.

Herbs

- Apply distilled **witch hazel** with cotton wool, then apply **calendula** (marigold) cream. **Tea tree** and **lavender essential oil** are antiseptic and can be added to the cream (1 drop per 10 ml of cream) or the drawing mixture below.

- **Slippery elm** powder can be mixed with **marshmallow root** powder or **comfrey root** powder and hot water to make a paste which can be applied to the boils to draw them.

- **Echinacea** is antiseptic and stimulates the immune system. **Wild indigo** is an anti-infective remedy, especially useful where the condition is persistent. Take them together as a decoction, using 1 to 2 tsp per cup, 2 to 3 times a day.

- **Cleavers** and **marigold** both help to clear the lymphatic tissue so have an infusion of 1 to 2 tsp per cup 3 times a day. **Blue flag** stimulates the lymph, circulation and bowels.

- **Burdock** is a very efficient tissue cleanser. Either of these can be made as a decoction using $\frac{1}{2}$ tsp per cup to take 2 to 3 times a day.

- **Nettles** are nutritious and cleansing and can be taken as an infusion of 1 to 2 tsp per cup 2 to 3 times a day. Ideally, add some warming herb to your brew, such as a few grains of **cayenne** powder or a little **ginger** to each cup.

Available products

Arkocaps' *Phytoderma* (burdock), *Phytokold* (echinacea).
Gerard's *Echinacea* or *Echinacea and Garlic* tablets, *Blue Flag Root Compound* tablets (with burdock and sarsaparilla).
Potter's *Skin Clear* tablets (echinacea), *Elixir of Echinacea* (also fumitory, wild indigo).

Bronchitis

Chest infections often follow a cold and can be difficult to clear. Repeated infections weaken the lungs, making them more prone to infection.

Smoking causes stagnation of the protective mucus of the lungs, so should be stopped.

Once infected, the mucus has to be coughed up or the infection will persist. Use an expectorant to do this and ask someone to bang on your back to dislodge the mucus. Deep breathing will also stimulate coughing and help to bring the mucus up. See *Asthma, Catarrh, Colds*, and *Convalescence* on page 13.

When to seek professional help

- If the condition is accompanied by difficulty in breathing, wheezing, fever or pain.

- Repeated bronchitis needs thorough investigation.

Diet and supplements

- Avoid dairy products.

- Garlic, horseradish and onions are antibiotic, so eat a plentiful amount.

- See *Catarrh* for a mucus-free diet.

Herbs

- **Thyme** is antiseptic to the lungs, and is expectorant and anti-spasmodic. **Elecampane** is a stimulating expectorant and anti-bacterial. **Horehound** is also a stimulating expectorant and **hyssop** is anti-spasmodic and expectorant. **Mullein** is a soothing expectorant where there is irritation and pain and is a tonic to inflamed mucous membranes. Make an infusion using 1 to 2 tsp per cup of the herb/s and drink freely. Add a few grains of **cayenne** powder to each cup.

- Take **coltsfoot** as an infusion of 1 to 2 tsp per cup or 1 tsp of the tincture 2 to 3 times a day to strengthen the lungs. Continue this for a few months if you continually suffer from bronchitis. As well as being a relaxing expectorant, it is high in zinc and is healing to the lung tissue.

- Essential oils of **eucalyptus, hyssop, tea tree, thyme, pine** and **wintergreen** can be used in a chest rub and applied to the chest and back. Use 10 drops of essential oil in 10 to 20 ml of vegetable oil. You can also use the oils in a vapouriser or oil burner to ease breathing. Add 10 drops of essential oil to the bath or to a bowl of hot water for a steam inhalation to relieve congestion.

Available products

Arkocaps' *Phytocoff* (thyme), *Phytokold* (echinacea), *Phytoseptik* (eucalyptus). Gerard's *Iceland Moss Compound* (also liquorice, lobelia) and *Echinacea & Garlic* tablets.
Potter's *Vegetable Cough Remover* (includes lobelia, elecampane, horehound, hyssop), *Antifect* (garlic, echinacea), *Horehound and Aniseed Cough Mixture* (includes elecampane, horehound, lobelia), *Antibron* tablets (includes lobelia, wild lettuce, coltsfoot), *Chest Mixture No. 80* (includes horehound, lobelia), *Special Cough Mixture* (liquorice, coltsfoot, euphorbia, elecampane), *Succus Allii* (garlic).
Allen's and Co. *Coltsfoot, Pine and Honey Cough Mixture.*
Olbas oil and pastilles are very widely available.

Candidiasis/Candida

Candida albicans, otherwise known as *thrush*, is a yeast-like fungus that can proliferate in the intestines, mouth and/or vagina, when the environment is favourable.

It is a common problem in diabetes and pregnancy, and in conditions where the immune system is suppressed, for example AIDS. It can occur as a result of taking antibiotics, immuno-suppressant drugs, the contraceptive pill or steroids.

The long list of symptoms includes allergies, bloating, constipation, cystitis, depression, diarrhoea, fatigue and headaches.

Oral thrush appears as white spots on the tongue and the inside of the mouth. It can become sore and cause a burning sensation.

Candida is very much a problem of our times. The typical western diet of white sugar, refined carbhydrates and fast food is largely to blame. See *Athlete's foot, Constipation, Thrush.*

When to seek professional help

Make sure candida really is your problem, especially before embarking on a very restricted diet.

Diet and supplements

- Sugar, in any form, refined carbohydrates and alcohol should be avoided with any fungal infection, whichever part of the body is afflicted.

- For intestinal candida, and entrenched candida infection elsewhere in the body, avoid yeast-containing foods and drinks, such as bread, cheese, mushrooms, yeast-based spreads, soya sauce, vinegar and all other fermented foods, unpeeled and dried fruit, fruit juices and shelled nuts. In severe cases avoid fruit and milk, which also contain sugars.

- Milk products in general, apart from live yoghurt, are fermented and contain yeast.

- Avoid any supplements containing yeast, and meat that has been intensively reared using antibiotics, steroids and hormones.

- Eat plenty of fresh vegetables, especially **garlic** (2 to 3 raw cloves a day) and onions, as they have anti-fungal properties.

- Olive oil (cold-pressed) is anti-fungal. Have 2 to 3 tbsp per day and use it raw on salads.

- **Cinnamon** has anti-fungal properties and can be included in the diet, where appropriate.

- Fresh pineapple can be very effective against oral thrush.

- Live natural yoghurt (100 g minimum) or Acidophilus, as Superdophilus, or Probion should be taken daily to promote the growth of beneficial bacteria in the digestive system.

- **Note:** The fungus dies off when it is deprived of its sugary diet, and it is common to feel worse initially.

Herbs

- **Marigold**, **rosemary** and **thyme** possess anti-fungal properties and can be taken as a tea. Infuse 1 to 2 tsp per cup 2 to 3 times a day. For oral thrush a double strength brew of any of these herbs can be made to use as a gargle 2 to 4 times a day, with 1 to 2 drops of **tea tree essential oil** added to each cup of gargle.

- **Pau d'Arco** (the bark of the South American taheebo tree) is an anti-fungal agent and is available as a tea from some health food shops.

- **Echinacea** root can be taken to stimulate the immune system. Take a decoction of 1 to 2 tsp per cup 1 to 3 times a day.

- **Tea tree** oil is a very effective anti-fungal agent. It is available as pessaries/suppositories which can be inserted into the rectum at night, if candida is present in the digestive tract.

Available products

Arkocaps' *Phytokold* (echinacea).
Gerard's *Echinacea* or *Echinacea and Garlic* tablets.
House of Mistry's *Tea Tree Oil Pessaries*.
Potter's *Antifect* (garlic and echinacea).

Catarrh

Mucus is necessary to protect the tissues from the environment. However, production can become excessive, and then is associated with inflamed mucous membranes. The cause can be related to diet, or congestion in the respiratory system, perhaps because of a cold. It can signify general congestion and overload in the body, possibly due to digestive weakness.

Irritants include smoking, so this should be stopped if a cure is to be achieved. See *Allergies, Asthma, Bronchitis, Colds, Sinusitis.*

Diet and supplements

- Avoid all dairy products, sugar and refined carbohydrates, as they are mucus forming.

- Avoid coffee, tea, chocolate, cocoa and cola drinks and all junk food.

- Eat something raw before each meal, as this tones the mucous membranes and boosts the body's powers of elimination.

- Include onions, and raw **garlic**, a clove a day, in your daily diet.

- Lemon, grapefruit and apple cider vinegar (up to 3 tbsp per day, with water and honey to taste) all help to clear mucus out of the system.

- Consider the Hay diet (see page 30). See also *What is a healthy diet?* on page 25.

Herbs

- For upper respiratory catarrh, **eyebright**, **elderflowers** and **ribwort** are very effective. Any of these can be taken as an infusion using 1 to 2 tsp per cup 2 to 3 times a day.

- **Golden seal** is an excellent tonic to the mucous membranes, especially where the problem is chronic. Have an infusion of $\frac{1}{4}$ to $\frac{1}{2}$ tsp of the powdered herb per cup 2 to 3 times a day. (It should not be taken during pregnancy or with high blood pressure, nor used long-term without the advice of a medical herbalist).

- Bitter remedies are helpful where toxins are contributing to the congestion, and where the mucous membranes are hot and inflamed. **Burdock**, **dandelion** root or **gentian** might be used.

- Where the condition is related to a sluggish metabolism and poor circulation, herbs like **cayenne**, **cinnamon**, **ginger** and **horseradish** can be used.

- **Echinacea** is appropriate where there is an infective element.

Available products

Gerard's *Echinacea* or *Echinacea and Garlic* tablets.
Potter's *Antifect* tablets (garlic and echinacea), *Catarrh Mixture* (boneset, blue flag, burdock, hyssop, capsicum).

Chilblains

These are painful patches of inflamed, swollen tissue usually found on the feet or hands. They itch and burn, and can become ulcerated. They are caused by poor circulation, so the blood flow needs to be encouraged into these tissues. See *Circulatory problems*.

Herbs

- **Cayenne** powder can be sprinkled into socks or tights before putting them on. In the form of **capsicum** tincture it can be applied neat to unbroken chilblains.

- If the skin has broken, bathe chilblains in an infusion of **comfrey leaf** and **marigold** flowers to speed healing.

- **Calendula** (marigold) and **comfrey** ointment can also be applied.

Cholesterol

Cholesterol has received something of a bad press over recent years but it is actually vital to good health. It is produced by the body and is present in every cell. As one example, cholesterol is vital in the formation of bile which is necessary for digestion.

The problem with cholesterol lies in the risk of it being deposited on the artery walls while it is in transit in the bloodstream.

Fatty foods undoubtedly raise cholesterol levels, but it is the type and quality of the fat being ingested that is of significance.

Fats are very susceptible to the effects of heat, light and air, and easily become rancid. Rancid fat is detrimental to health, and is associated with arteriosclerosis. The majority of available vegetable oils are refined using heat and chemicals and these same oils are further processed to make margarine. They are hydrogenated in order to make them solid, a process which causes them to raise cholesterol levels.

A diet high in sugar, refined carbohydrates and refined fats (any of which might be found in processed and pre-packaged foods) is a major culprit in the incidence of heart disease.

Stress is another factor. It can affect the efficiency of the digestive system and its metabolism of fats by the liver.

The negative effects of smoking must not be forgotten.

Animal and vegetable fat has to undergo the same breakdown processes in the body, but only animal products actually contain cholesterol. A very low fat or cholesterol-free diet is indicated where there is severe arteriosclerosis and heart disease. This might also be indicated for hypercholesterolaemia (excess cholesterol in the blood, often due to hereditary factors) until the condition is stabilised. The longer the blood levels of cholesterol are raised the greater the risk of arteriosclerosis. A modification of the diet and the types of fat being eaten is often the only action required to lower the levels. See *Arteriosclerosis*.

When to seek professional help

- If cholesterol levels are high – above 7 mmol/litre (kits for measuring cholesterol are available).

- If there is associated arteriosclerosis and heart disease.

- If there is a family history of high cholesterol or heart disease.

Exercise

- Walking, a couple of miles a day if you can manage it, or any exercise which is enjoyable, is of benefit.

- Exposure to sunshine helps.

Diet and supplements

- Avoid refined vegetable oils and margarine.

- Use only cold-pressed (virgin) oils such as olive, safflower and sunflower.

- Heat is detrimental to the nature of all fats, especially at high temperatures. Fat should never be heated until it bubbles or burns, so deep fat frying should be avoided. The re-heating of fat for frying is positively toxic. It is always preferable to grill.

- Fish oils reduce cholesterol levels in the blood. Eat oily fish like mackerel or take fish oils in liquid or capsule form.

- Vitamin C is important in mobilising cholesterol. Pectin found in fruit is also important, so eat plenty of fresh fruit, especially apples.

- Vegetables are essential. Especially beneficial are **garlic**, onions, alfalfa, asparagus, chickpeas, fenugreek, lentils, soya and spinach.

- Foods containing fibre reduce cholesterol levels and oats have been shown to be very effective.

- Vitamin E, found in wheatgerm, helps protect against arteriosclerosis.
- Lecithin is very effective in lowering blood cholesterol. It is present in foods like soya beans, and can be obtained in capsule or granule form.
- Live yoghurt helps reduce cholesterol levels.
- **Evening primrose oil** can be taken as a supplement. It contains the essential fatty acids important in protecting against arteriosclerosis.
- Avoid commercially produced products like roasted nuts and peanut butter (which contains hydrogenated oils unless otherwise stated).
- Avoid coffee, caffeinated and decaffeinated.

Herbs

- **Dandelion** root stimulates the breakdown of fat by the liver. Have a decoction of 1 to 2 tsp per cup 2 to 3 times a day.
- **Garlic**, already mentioned under diet, reduces the amount of fat and cholesterol in the blood. It needs to be taken long-term to prove effective. Eat 2 to 3 almond-sized cloves of **garlic** daily, in salad dressings and cooking or take the **garlic capsules** which are now widely available.

Circulatory problems (poor circulation)

Poor circulation most commonly shows itself as cold hands and feet but can result in a more general feeling of coldness. Exercise does not necessarily relieve the situation. It is not uncommon for the lips and extremities to turn blue with cold. Poor circulation will contribute to congestion in the body. See *Arteriosclerosis, Chilblains, Varicose veins*.

When to seek professional help

- If the condition is deteriorating and not responding to the suggestions below.
- If it is associated with heart problems or arteriosclerosis.

Exercise

- Walking, simple keep-fit, swimming and running all help to get the circulation flowing.

Diet and supplements

- Blue and black fruit such as plums, blackberries, blueberries, dark cherries and blackcurrants provide bioflavonoids, which are important for the integrity of the blood vessel walls. Buckwheat is also high in bioflavonoids, notably rutin. Rutin can be taken in tablet form. Take 6 per day.

Herbs

- A **mustard** foot bath is an effective way to stimulate the circulation. Use 1 tbsp of the powder per bowl of hot water. **Cayenne** or **ginger** might be used instead, but use half the amount of cayenne.

- **Horseradish** is a circulatory stimulant and will improve the circulation. The plain grated root can be obtained from greengrocers. Use 1 tsp 1 to 2 times a day sprinkled on food or in a dressing.

- **Prickly ash** bark also improves blood flow. Make a decoction of 1 tsp per cup to take 2 to 3 times a day.

- **Cayenne** also stimulates the circulation. Use the tip of a teaspoon 2 to 3 times a day, added to a tea, or your meal.

Available products

Arkocaps' *Phytotravel* (ginger).
Gerard's *Prickly Ash* tablets.

Colds

Colds tend to strike when your resistance is low, perhaps due to tiredness, depression or stress. They are most common in winter, when diets tend to be lacking in fresh (raw) fruit and vegetables, which provide vitamin C, and high in starchy foods, which congest the system. Colds can be alleviated but should not be suppressed, as they are a cleansing process. Try not to carry on regardless but listen to your body and make sure you get a good night's sleep. The herbal approach is to aid the body in dealing with the virus and eliminate the toxic waste. See *Catarrh, Coughs, Influenza, Sore throat.*

Diet and supplements

- Avoid all dairy products, sugar and refined carbohydrates to prevent excess mucus production and to help the immune system.

- Try to stick mainly to fruit and vegetables, or even fast for 1 to 2 days on juices (see page 12).

- **Garlic** and onions are anti-infective, and are most beneficial raw.

- Vitamin C boosts the immune system. Take this as a supplement of 500 mg to 1 g per day.

Herbs

- **Elderflowers**, **peppermint** and **yarrow** are excellent to have as an infusion, ideally at the first sign of a cold. This mixture will promote the circulation and relieve congestion. Use 1 to 2 tsp per cup and drink freely. Honey and lemon juice can be added to taste. A slice of fresh, or a pinch of dried **ginger**, **cinnamon** or **cayenne**, can be added to each cup for extra effectiveness.

- **Mustard** foot baths really are effective. Use 1 tbs of **mustard** powder per bowl or bucket of boiling water. Place your feet in the water, as hot as you can bear. The water level should be well above the ankles. Soak your feet for about 10 minutes, then retire to bed and keep warm.

Available products

Arkocaps' *Phytokold* (echinacea), *Phytoseptik* (eucalyptus).
Gerard's *Echinacea and Garlic* tablets.
Potter's *Peerless Composition Essence* (includes capsicum and prickly ash), *Life Drops* (capsicum, elderflowers, peppermint), *Elderflowers, Peppermint with Composition Essence, Antifect* (garlic, echinacea).

Cold sores

These skin lesions are caused by the herpes simplex virus, which remains latent in the nervous system after the initial infection and re-emerges when the immune system is compromised. This usually happens when we are stressed physically, mentally or emotionally. Cold sores can also appear on exposure to extremes of temperature, for example with sunburn. Treatment involves boosting the immune and the nervous systems. See *Stress*.

Diet and supplements

- Dietary changes are important in raising the level of resistance to the virus. See *What is a healthy diet?* on page 25.

Herbs

- **Echinacea** stimulates the immune system and a decoction of 1 tsp per cup should be drunk freely as soon as the cold sore begins to tingle. Alternatively, take it in tablet form, taking one every 2 to 3 hours.

- **Lemon balm** has anti-viral properties, as well as being uplifting and relaxing. Make an infusion using 1 tsp per cup. It can be drunk freely and also dabbed on to the cold sore.

- Tinctures of **golden seal**, **marigold** or **myrrh** can be dabbed on to the lesion.

- **St John's wort oil** or **garlic oil** (see page 19) might be applied. Essential oils of **lavender** or **melissa (lemon balm)** might be added to any of the above. Use 1 drop of essential oil per 1 ml of tincture or oil. Apply at least 3 times a day to the lesion.

Available products

Arkocaps' *Phytokold* (echinacea).
Gerard's *Echinacea* or *Echinacea and Garlic* tablets.
Potter's *Antifect* (garlic and echinacea).

Colitis

This is an umbrella term meaning inflammation of the colon, incorporating such conditions as irritable bowel syndrome and ulcerative colitis. Infection, food intolerance, anxiety and stress are all factors to be taken into consideration. If there is also diverticular disease the recommended diet is different. See *Allergies*, *Anxiety*, *Constipation*, *Diarrhoea*, *Stress*.

When to seek professional help

If you suffer from colitis you need to see a medical herbalist. The condition is complex and varies in severity. There can be violent diarrhoea, blood and/or mucus loss, and weight loss. Correct diagnosis is vital.

Diet and supplements

- Dairy products and wheat are most commonly implicated if the cause is a food intolerance, so it is worth experimenting by cutting one or both out of the diet completely for at least 1 or 2 weeks.

- A bland diet will not irritate the inflamed mucous membranes of the colon, so fibre is best avoided initially. Eat well-cooked root vegetables, mashed potatoes, white bread, flour and rice.

- **Garlic** is specific for any infection in the gut, although it is not always well tolerated.

Herbs

- Herbs that might be indicated include those to astringe the diarrhoea, blood or mucus, such as **bistort**, **tormentil** and **witch hazel**.

- **Chamomile**, **comfrey leaf**, **marigold**, **marshmallow root**, **meadowsweet** and **slippery elm** are healing and soothing.

- **Golden seal** is an excellent tonic to the mucous membranes.

Available products

Gerard's *Cranesbill* tablets, *Fenulin* tablets (fenugreek, slippery elm, hydrastis), *Golden Seal Compound* tablets (also marshmallow root, cranesbill, dandelion root).

Conjunctivitis

This is inflamation of the protective membrane of the eye, caused by infection, an allergy (like hay fever) or a foreign body (such as an eyelash) or chemicals in the eye. The whites of the eye become pink or red, are sore and irritate. Where there is an infection, they can become weepy, with the eyelids sticking together after sleep. Care must be taken not to spread the infection to the other eye or to other members of the family.

When to seek professional help

Eyes are delicate organs. Make sure of the diagnosis, as eye conditions can deteriorate rapidly. Warning signs include accompanying pain, headache, visual disturbance or swelling.

Herbs

- A sore inflamed eye can be soothed with an eyewash using equal parts of **eyebright** and **calendula**. A few grains of salt can be added to each eyebathful. Do this 2 to 3 times a day. A fresh mixture should be made up every day.

- Alternatively, dilute 1 part distilled **witch hazel** in 3 to 5 parts boiled water to use in an eyebath.

Constipation

Ideally there should be at least one bowel movement per day to clear the body of toxins. Diet is the biggest cause of constipation but consider any drugs that are being taken or food intolerance. The bowel can be too slow and slack or the bowel can be too tight and cannot let the faeces move through freely.

Tension commonly contributes to the condition, with diarrhoea alternating with constipation at times of stress. When this happens laxatives should not be used – the condition needs to be treated with relaxants.

Constipation can also be a result of laxative abuse or come after taking antibiotics. Laxatives should not be used as a matter of course as the bowel can become dependent on them and lose its tone. Laxative abuse will also lead to nutritional deficiences. See *Allergies, Anxiety, Bilious attack, Colitis, Stress*.

When to seek professional help

- If the onset is sudden, or accompanied by blood in the stools.

- If laxatives are the only effective way of dealing with the problem, despite dietary changes.

Exercise

This is important to main bowel motility. Constipation is commonly attributed to a sedentary lifestyle. It is also important to obey the urge to defaecate.

Diet and supplements

- Maintain a good fibre intake of green vegetables, potatoes with their skins, wholewheat flour, bread, pasta and brown rice.

- Dried and fresh fruit help combat constipation, especially apricots, figs and prunes.

- Cut out refined foods, tea, coffee (coffee is a stimulant to the gut but it can over-tense the bowel) and chocolate.

- Animal products can cause constipation, so assess your intake of meat and dairy produce.

- **Linseeds** are an excellent bulk laxative that can be taken long-term to promote adequate bowel movement. Sprinkle 1 tsp–1 tbs on your breakfast cereal, with at least $\frac{1}{4}$ to $\frac{1}{2}$ pint (150 to 300 ml) of liquid. This can be repeated later in the day if necessary. Porridge is also a bulk laxative. Linseeds and porridge are preferable to bran but if you have been using bran and it is the only thing that works, just make sure that you are not taking it with excessive sugar or buy a sugar-free alternative from a health food shop.

- Make sure you are drinking enough water, at least 1 to 2 litres per day.

Herbs

- **Psyllium seeds** improve the bulk of the stools – 2 tsp in a cup of water, left to soak for 15 minutes, forms a gel which can be taken morning and evening.

- **Dandelion root** is a gentle stimulant to the digestive system and laxative. Make a decoction using 1 tsp per cup 2 to 3 times a day.

- **Rhubarb root** is a stronger laxative so use half the dose.

- **Chamomile** is relaxing and has a specific action on the gut. Use an infusion of 1 to 2 tsp per cup 2 to 3 times a day where tension is a factor.

- **Cramp bark** can be taken as a decoction of 1 tsp per cup 1 to 2 times a day to relax the muscle walls of the bowel where there is tension and pain.

- **Chamomile**, **ginger**, **fennel** or **peppermint** help to deal with any griping or wind that accompany the effect of a strong laxative like **senna**. Infuse 1 tsp per cup of the herbs, $\frac{1}{2}$ tsp of crushed seed, or $\frac{1}{4}$ tsp of powdered **ginger**.

- **Ginger** is an excellent tonic to the bowel, especially for the elderly as loss of tone occurs with increasing years.

Available products

Arkocaps' *Phytofibre* (ispaghula – equivalent to psyllium), *Phytosenalax* (senna), *Phytotravel* (ginger).
Gerard's *Gladlax* tablets (aloes, valerian, fennel, holy thistle), *Priory Cleansing Herbs* (senna, buckthorn, fennel, psyllium).
Potter's *Cleansing Herb* (buckthorn, psyllium, senna), *Out of Sorts* tablets (senna, aloes, cascara, dandelion, fennel), *Senna* tablets.

Coughs

These can be due to infection, nervousness, an environmental irritant or prescription drugs. If you are taking any drug ask a qualified practitioner about the possibility of it causing the problem. For nervous coughs see *Anxiety* and *Stress*. Consider an allergy, see *Asthma*. See *Bronchitis, Catarrh, Colds, Sore throats*.

When to seek professional help

- If you start to cough up blood.
- If it is accompanied by chest pain, difficulty in breathing and/or fever.
- If the cough persists for more than two weeks.

Diet and supplements

- As with any infection or inflammation involving the mucous membranes you should avoid dairy products, sugar and refined carbohydrates, as these lead to excess mucus production and congestion.
- Eat **garlic** and onions for their antiseptic and expectorant properties.
- Honey and fresh lemon as a hot drink can be very soothing.

Herbs

- If colds have a tendency to go on to your chest, **coltsfoot** can be taken for a period of three months to strengthen the lungs. It is a soothing expectorant where there is irritaton and a nervous element to the cough. An infusion of 1 tsp per cup can be taken 1 to 3 times a day.
- **Wild cherry bark** can be taken for an irritated, unproductive, nervous cough. Have a decoction of 1 tsp per cup 2 to 3 times a day.
- See *Bronchitis* for herbs to deal with infection.

Cramp

This painful contraction of muscle most commonly occurs in the calves and at night. It is particularly common in the last three months of pregnancy, due to the increased demand for calcium. Apart from a lack of calcium, cramp is also associated with poor circulation. See *Circulatory problems*.

Exercise

If you have an attack of cramp, stand at arm's length from a wall, place your palms flat against the wall and lean into it with your feet flat on the floor.

Diet and supplements

- Eat plenty of calcium-rich foods, such as green leafy vegetables, almonds and sesame seeds (tahini is the pulped seeds).
- Too much protein in the diet causes a loss of calcium from the body, so assess the amount of meat and dairy produce in your diet.

- Absorption of calcium is dependent on there being enough stomach acidity and the presence of vitamin D (found in sunlight and fish oils), magnesium and a small amount of fat.

- A calcium and magnesium supplement can prove helpful.

Herbs

- **Cramp bark** is a muscle relaxant. A decoction using 1 tsp per cup can be taken 1 to 2 times a day.

- **Rosemary essential oil** stimulates the circulation. Put 10 drops in 10 ml of base oil and massage in vigorously during an attack.

Available products

Gerard's *Cramp Bark* tablets.

Cystitis

This inflammation of the bladder is most frequently caused by an infection and is more likely to affect women than men. Symptoms include frequent urination accompanied by a burning sensation. The infection can spread up the tubules to the kidneys, causing a kidney infection.

Prolonged use of antibiotics can exacerbate the condition, as the bacteria tend to become resistant to the treatment. See *Allergies, Candidiasis, Prostate problems*.

When to seek professional help

- If the symptoms of cystitis do not improve within a few days.

- If you are passing blood.

- If you are suffering from low back pain, a temperature, headache and generally feel unwell.

- If you are pregnant.

Diet and supplements

- It is important to drink plenty of fluids with cystitis – several pints (1 to 2 litres) of water per day. Barley water can be made by simmering 1 oz (25 g) of barley in 1 pint (500 ml) of water for 20 minutes. Cranberry juice (sugar-free) is also helpful.

- Have plenty of fresh fruit and vegetables. Onions, leeks and **garlic** are particularly therapeutic.

- Avoid sugar, alcohol, caffeine and red meat.

Herbs

- **Corn silk** or **marshmallow** herb will help to soothe cystitis. Have an infusion of 1 tsp per cup 2 to 3 times a day.

- **Couchgrass** is soothing and anti-microbial. Have a decoction using 1 to 2 tsp per cup 2 to 3 times a day.

- **Buchu** is antiseptic to the urinary system. Have an infusion of 1 tsp per cup 2 to 3 times a day. A decoction of **echinacea** could alternatively be used.

- **Horsetail** can be taken during cystitis. It is generally strengthening to the urinary system. Have an infusion of 1 tsp per cup 1 to 2 times a day.

- **Parsley piert** has a restorative effect on the kidneys and is helpful if there is a history of kidney problems. Have an infusion using 1 to 2 tsp per cup 1 to 3 times a day.

- **Dandelion herb** can be used as a diuretic to help flush the toxins out of the body. Have as an infusion of 1 to 2 tsp per cup 2 to 3 times a day.

Available products

Arkocaps' *Phytosistisus* (cherry stalks), *Phytokold* (echinacea).
Gerard's *Buchu Compound* tablets (buchu, dandelion root, uva-ursi, cleavers), *Echinacea* tablets, *Herbal Powder No. 8* (dandelion leaf, uva-ursi, couchgrass, buchu), *Waterlex* tablets (dandelion root, horsetail, uva-ursi), *Garlic* tablets.
Potter's *Antitis* tablets (buchu, cleavers, couchgrass, horsetail, shepherd's purse, uva-ursi), *Infusion of Buchu Concentrated, Infusion of Uva Ursi Concentrated* or *Diuretabs* (buchu, juniper, parsley piert, uva ursi), *Garlic* tablets.

Dandruff

The skin of the scalp is shed like anywhere else on the body but this natural sloughing-off of skin cells can become excessive and cause distress.

The scales associated with dandruff are rarely due to an isolated problem and should be viewed as a skin condition, in which diet plays an important role. Excessive oil production from the glands in the scalp is a common factor, with the presence of a bacterial or fungal element.

Avoid using harsh, medicated shampoos. Something mild, like a baby shampoo or the ones suggested below are more appropriate. See *Acne, Eczema.*

Diet and supplements

- See *What is a healthy diet?* on page 25.

Herbs

- Use an infusion, 1 oz (25 g) per ½ pint (250 ml), of a mixture of **burdock root** (ground), **nettles** and **rosemary** as a hair rinse (cooled) and massage into the scalp every other day after shampooing. This is stimulating and nutritive to the scalp.

- **Rosemary oil** might also be used, perhaps with **tea tree oil** which has antifungal and antiseptic properties. Use 10 drops of essential oil per 10 ml of olive oil (antifungal) and massage into the scalp. Leave on overnight and wash the hair in the morning. See *Acne* and *Eczema* for internal remedies.

Available products

Cornucopia's *Nettle and Lavender, Rosemary and Lime, Tea Tree and Lemon* shampoos.
Neal's Yard and Weleda shampoos.
Potter's *Adiantine* (southernwood, bay oil, rosemary oil, witch hazel) or *Medicated Extract of Rosemary Bay Rum*.

Depression

This can be the result of chronic tiredness, emotional upset due to bereavement or the break-up of a relationship, or when there is a loss of identity and purpose in life. It can also be due to vitamin or mineral deficiency, food intolerance, hormonal imbalance, illness or a liver disorder. It has also been linked to the lack of daylight during the winter months, so if your depression if seasonal, or you work or live in conditions with very little daylight, use daylight simulation bulbs and try to change your environment to allow in more natural light. See *Allergies, Anxiety, Stress, Premenstrual tension*.

When to seek professional help

- If you are taking orthodox drugs, such as anti-depressants and tranquillisers.

- If the condition is severe.

- If you would like to talk to a counsellor.

Exercise

- Fresh air and exercise is always beneficial.

- Dancing, singing and music can all help enormously.

Diet and supplements

Follow a wheat-free diet (see page 29) if wheat is found to be the cause of the depression, otherwise follow the dietary advice given under *Stress*.

Herbs

- **Borage**, **lavender**, **lemon balm** and **rosemary** are all relaxing and uplifting tonics.

- **St John's wort**, **skullcap** and **vervain** are restorative and calming. Any of these herbs can be made up as an infusion, using 1 to 2 tsp per cup 3 times a day.

Diarrhoea

This is the body's attempt to expel an irritant from the bowel. Causes include infection, food poisoning and intestinal parasites. Antibiotics, especially broad-spectrum ones, can cause diarrhoea. They upset the balance of the gut flora as they are non-selective in which bacteria they destroy. Other drugs might be implicated.

Diarrhoea is also a symptom of colitis, Crohn's disease and irritable bowel syndrome.

Stress can be a factor, causing over-stimulation of the bowel.

Chronic diarrhoea can also be a sign of a food allergy, commonly due to milk or wheat. See *Allergies, Colitis*.

When to seek professional help

- If the diarrhoea does not improve within 24 to 36 hours.

- If it is particularly violent, and accompanied by severe pain, vomiting, a high temperature or blood loss.

- Babies and young children need special attention as they easily become dehydrated.

Diet and supplements

- Maintaining fluid levels is most important.

- Dioralyte, which can be obtained from a chemist, will replace lost fluids and salts. Alternatively, drink one part apple, grape or orange juice diluted with three parts of fresh water, with a pinch of salt added to it.

- Rice or barley water is excellent. Boil 1 oz (25 g) rice or barley in 1 pint (500 ml) water till cooked, strain the water off and drink it.

- It is best not to eat until the diarrhoea has stopped, then start with vegetable juices, fruit and steamed vegetables.

- Live yoghurt or acidophylus tablets will help to re-establish the gut flora and get the digestive system back to normal quickly.

Herbs

The idea is to help the body deal with the causative agent without suppressing the gut from expelling any toxins (morphine-based products stop the bowel from moving).

- **Garlic** is effective against pathogenic bacteria in the gut, while selectively sparing the beneficial flora. Up to 4 to 6 cloves per day can be taken, either crushed and swallowed in water, or added to some vegetable juice or live yoghurt.

- **Echinacea** as a decoction of 1 to 2 tsp per cup can be drunk freely as an anti-microbial agent and to boost the immune system.

- **Chamomile** and/or **peppermint** will help to soothe and settle the digestive system.

- **Meadowsweet** is soothing and anti-inflammatory. Infusions of 1 to 2 tsp per cup of these herbs can be taken freely.

- **Slippery elm** as powder or tablets will soothe a sore gut.

- Astringents, like **bistort root**, **tormentil root** and **witch hazel** (not the distilled variety), have their place in the treatment of acute, short-term diarrhoea. They are best used after all the faeces have been evacuated. The tannins in these herbs bind with the gut wall, creating a barrier to organisms and toxins. They quell irritation and inflammation and so slow down the movement of the bowel. Make a decoction of $\frac{1}{2}$ to 1 tsp per cup and add honey for taste. A pinch of **cinnamon** can be added to each cup of tea. Apart from improving flavour, it contains tannins and is a calming and warming digestive tonic.

- Strong black tea could be used as an astringent, if nothing else is on hand.

Available products

Gerard's *Cranesbill* tablets.
Potter's *Spanish Tummy Mixture* (blackberry root bark, cathecu).

Earache

Pain is most commonly caused by an infection or inflammation occurring in the middle or outer ear. It can also be due to referred pain from the teeth.

Babies and young children are particularly prone to ear infections, as their relatively short eustachian tube easily becomes blocked if there is a catarrhal infection. Excessive secretion of wax is a sign of an unresolved infection or a catarrhal problem.

Antibiotics are not the answer for recurrent ear infections and trials have demonstrated that they have no positive effect on the resolution of the condition. See *Catarrh*, *Fever*, and *Ear infections* under *Children*.

When to seek professional help

- If the problem is recurrent.
- If the eardrum is perforated.
- If there is bleeding or discharge.
- If you suspect a middle ear infection.

Action

Hot salt packs can ease the pain considerably. Find a cotton or muslin bag big enough to comfortably cover the ear and the surrounding area. Half-fill it with hot, dry salt (heat the salt in a saucepan or oven). When it is just cool enough to hold against the ear, do so, keeping it there until it cools off.

Diet and supplements

See *Catarrh*.

Herbs

- **Garlic**, **mullein** or **St John's wort oil**, preferably warmed, see page 19, make excellent ear drops. Put 2 drops in each ear (even if only one ear is hurting). **Lavender essential oil** might be added to any of the above. Use 1 drop of essential oil per 1 ml of base oil for added effect. **Myrrh oil** could also be used. Tinctures of **Pasque flower** or **lobelia** (which needs to be prescribed by a medical herbalist) to help relieve the pain can be added to any of the above at the rate of 1 drop of tincture per ml of base oil. It is also useful to include **golden seal** tincture where there is a middle ear infection.

- If the eardrum has perforated **do not** use eardrops; instead put the oil on a piece of cotton wool and place that in the ear. A boiled clove of **garlic** or piece of boiled onion can be placed in the ear if nothing else is on hand.

- Inhalations of essential oils like **eucalyptus**, **tea tree** and **thyme**, which are antiseptic, are useful. Add 10 drops of oil to a bowl of steaming hot water, and cover the head with a towel.

- **Echinacea**, as a decoction of 1 tsp per cup, tincture, 5–10 drops, or tablet, should be taken every hour.

- The internal remedies suggested under *Catarrh* can be used.

- Refer to *Fever*, if appropriate.

Eczema

This is inflammation of the skin that can be triggered by an internal or external irritant. External causes include detergents, skin products and jewellery (nickel). Hereditary, dietary and emotional factors can all play their part. Treatment involves assessing all the factors involved. Internal remedies are vital, with external ones being used to soothe not suppress. The skin can be viewed as a reflection of the nervous system. See *Allergies*, *Anxiety*, *Stress*.

When to seek professional help

Eczema tends to be a complex condition requiring individual treatment which is best undertaken with a medical herbalist, especially when steroid creams are being used. Eczema can become seriously infected.

Diet and supplements

- The diet suggested under *Asthma* can be applied here.

- Cold-pressed oils, like olive, safflower and sunflower, should be included in your diet. These supply the essential fatty acids vital for the health of the skin and the nervous system.

- **Linseed** oil is also an excellent source of fatty acids and can also be applied to the skin.

- Take **evening primrose oil** as capsules or use externally.

Herbs

- Distilled **witch hazel** is soothing and cooling. Dab it on with cotton wool.

- **Chamomile**, **chickweed** or **marigold** cream can be used to soothe the irritation.

- A bran bath can be used to soothe inflamed skin, especially if there is a large area. Put 6 oz (150 g) of bran into a cotton or muslin bag, soak this in the water and squeeze the bag well to release the resulting emolient liquid.

- Internal measures might include **nettles**, which are particularly effective where there is a strong allergic element. They are also a blood cleanser and nutritive. An infusion of 1 to 2 tsp per cup can be taken 2 to 3 times a day.

- **Cleavers** is also a tissue cleanser, specifically for the lymphatic system. Make up as for **nettles**.

- **Dandelion root** is a liver tonic that helps the body eliminate the toxins which can cause the inflammation. Have a decoction using 1 tsp per cup 2 to 3 times a day.

- **Burdock root** is also extremely effective but much more potent, so use half the dose.

Available products

Arkocaps *Phytofluid* (nettles), *Phytoderma* (burdock).

Fever

This should be carefully monitored but not suppressed, unless it becomes dangerously high. A raised temperature is the body's way of destroying the organism causing the infection. Sweating helps to clear out the toxins and regulate the temperature. See *Influenza*, and under *Children*.

When to seek professional help

- If the fever doesn't break within 2 to 3 days, or is recurrent.
- If a high temperature can't be brought under control.
- If the temperature drops, then sharply rises again.
- If a young child has a fever.

Action

If the temperature reaches 40°C (104°F), cool the body down with a tepid bath, or sponge-down with tepid water. Make sure there is enough ventilation in the room and clothing is light. A temperature is dangerous if it reaches 41°C (106°F) because brain damage can occur.

Diet

It is best to fast while you have a fever (you are unlikely to feel like eating anyway) but make sure you have plenty of liquids in the form of herb teas, pure water and diluted fruit juices.

Herbs

- **Boneset, elderflowers, ginger, hyssop, limeflowers, peppermint** and **yarrow** are all diaphoretic – that is they promote sweating during a fever. A mixture of any of these can be made into an infusion using 1 to 2 tsp per cup. This should be drunk freely with a fever.

- **Ginger** can be used fresh by crushing 2 to 3 slices in a garlic crusher and adding it to each cup. Alternatively, add the tip of a teaspoon to each cup of brew. For its anti-infective properties, crushed raw **garlic** can be added to, or swallowed with the herbs.

- A decoction of **echinacea**, 1 tsp per cup, should be sipped at regular intervals, or take 5 to 10 drops of the tincture or a tablet every hour. This is also anti-infective and will boost the body's defences.

- Sometimes a fever needs some impetus (a slight temperature can be boosted). Warming herbs include **echinacea**, **garlic** and **ginger**, and also **cayenne** (very stimulating) and **cinnamon**.

- **Catmint** will cool you down. Make an infusion with 1 tsp per cup and drink freely.

- Bitters like **dandelion root** and **gentian** are also cooling.

Available products

Arkocaps' *Phytokold* (echinacea), *Phytotravel* (ginger).
Gerard's *Echinacea*, and *Echinacea and Garlic* tablets.
Potter's *Antifect* (garlic and echinacea), *Peerless Composition Essence* (includes prickly ash, capsicum), *Life Drops* (capsicum, elderflowers, peppermint), *Elderflowers, Peppermint with Composition Essence*.

Gout

Gout is caused by an accumulation of uric acid crystals in the joints, most commonly the big toe, but it can also affect the ankles, knees, hands and feet. It can be excrutiatingly painful, with swelling and inflammation of the affected joint/s. Attacks are associated with high levels of uric acid in the system (see *Diet and supplements* below) and are commonly precipitated by surgery, alcohol, drugs, a high purine diet (see *Diet and supplements* below) and illness. Being overweight and having a high protein diet increases the likelihood of an attack.

Chronic gout is associated with kidney disease.

Treatment involves introducing a low purine diet to reduce the amount of uric acid being produced, using herbs to promote the excretion of uric acid from the body and tonifying the organs responsible for elimination. See *Kidney stones*, *Osteoarthritis* and *Rheumatism and Arthritis*.

When to seek professional help

Treatment is best undertaken with a qualified herbalist, especially if you are taking orthodox drugs for the condition. It is vital to prevent kidney damage.

Exercise

For long-term benefit, exercise should be increased but not during an attack. This ensures a better circulation and the crystals do not have a chance to form.

Diet and supplements

- Purines are the waste products produced on the breakdown of animal proteins in the body. Uric acid is such a purine. Therefore meat should be avoided, especially offal (liver, kidney, etc.) and red meat, also fish, especially shellfish and rich, oily fish like sardines.

- Consumption of eggs and dairy produce, especially cheese, should be minimal.

- Avoid pickled and smoked foods, yeast extracts, tea and coffee, and alcohol.

- Foods to eat include artichokes (globe and Jerusalem), asparagus and all fresh vegetables. Red cherries help to dissolve uric acid crystals.

Herbs

- **Celery seeds** are specific for eliminating uric acid from the body. Drink an infusion of 1 to 2 tsp of freshly crushed seeds 3 times a day.

- **Birch** is anti-inflammatory and diuretic, and is particularly useful during an acute attack of gout. Drink an infusion of 1 to 2 tsp of the leaves per cup freely.

- **Parsley piert** is important as a support and a restorative to the kidneys. Have an infusion of 1 to 2 tsp per cup 2 to 3 times a day.

- **Milkthistle** and **dandelion root** support the liver. A decoction of 1 to 2 tsp per cup should be taken 2 to 3 times a day. Dandelion root is also diuretic so will help flush the uric acid out of the system.

- A circulatory stimulant such as **prickly ash** will promote the mobilisation and excretion of the uric acid. Make a decoction of the root using 1 tsp per cup and take this 2 to 3 times a day.

Gum disease (Gingivitis)

Gingivitis (swollen, bleeding and infected gums) is notoriously common. If left untreated, the condition will gradually deteriorate, setting up a focus of infection which is constantly releasing toxins into the body and taxing the immune system. A more violent gum infection is pyorrhoea which can rapidly undermine the stability of the teeth and make them loose. Hormonal changes, such as those which occur in pregnancy, can heighten the problem. See *Bad breath.*

When to seek professional help

Any gum problems warrant a visit to your dentist. If the condition is severe, seek treatment from a qualified herbalist.

Diet and supplements

- Hot salt-water can be very effective, as can bicarbonate of soda. When the gums are particularly sore, use 1 tsp of either in a tumbler of hot water as a mouthwash 1 to 3 times a day.

- Make sure your intake of vitamin C is adequate. Take it as a supplement of up to 1 g a day, especially if your intake of raw fruit and vegetables is poor.

Herbs

- **Rosemary**, **sage** and **thyme** can all be used as a mouthwash. Use an infusion of 2 to 3 tsp per cup at least twice a day.

- **Myrrh** is best used in tincture form. Add ½ tsp to the above mouthwash.

- Add a pinch of **cayenne** to each cup to stimulate the blood flow to the gums.

- Stronger astringents, such as **bistort** and **witch hazel bark**, can be made up as a decoction using 1 tsp per cup.

- **Echinacea root** can be used internally and externally to fight infection. Make a decoction with 1 to 2 tsp per cup to use as a mouthwash and then swallow. Do this 2 to 3 times a day.

- Essential oils of **eucalyptus**, **lavender**, **myrrh**, **rosemary**, **sage**, **tea tree** and **thyme** might be used in a mouthwash, either individually or as a mixture, by adding 1 to 2 drops in total to a tumbler of warm water.

- Regular treatment should be kept up for 2 weeks.

Available products

Weleda's *Gargle and Mouthwash* (includes krameria, myrrh, sage, lavender, eucalyptus, peppermint) and toothpastes (their *Krameria* toothpaste is excellent for gum problems).
Tom's of Maine toothpastes.
Caution – Do not swallow a mouthwash unless your practitioner has advised you to do so.

Haemorrhoids (Piles)

These protrusions, either in the anal canal, or around the rectum are caused by distended veins. They can be the result of constipation, and straining, liver congestion, or pregnancy and labour. They can become very sore and inflamed, bleed easily and itch. See *Constipation*, *Liver disorders*, *Varicose veins*.

When to seek professional help

- If the piles start to bleed heavily.
- If the condition doesn't improve.

Exercise

- Avoid sitting down for long periods as this will encourage blood to pool in the area.
- Pelvic floor exercises can be most helpful.

Diet and supplements

- It is important to avoid constipation (straining exerts more pressure on the veins), so include plenty of fibre in your diet, such as fruit, vegetables and grains.

Herbs

- An ordinary teabag brewed for 15 minutes and applied cold to the area will help to astringe the piles.

- **Distilled witch hazel** will soothe itching and inflammation, (it is not as astringent as other **witch hazel** preparations).

- **Comfrey** and **calendula** ointments are healing and anti-inflammatory.

- **Bistort, witch hazel bark** and **horsechestnut**, 2 tsp per cup as a decoction and applied to the area with a pad of cotton wool will help to astringe and tone the blood vessels. This mixture can be made up as a cream with tinctures and a syringe without the needle (consult a practitioner) can be used to inject the liquid or cream (5 to 10 ml) into the rectum.

- Ice-cubes could be made up of any of the liquid preparations and applied externally. Alternatively, use the plastic bag ice moulds and insert these into the rectum.

- Preparations should be used after each bowel movement, as required, or twice a day.

- **Dandelion root** can be taken when there is liver congestion and/or constipation. Have a decoction of 1 to 2 tsp per cup 1 to 2 times a day.

Available products

Arkocaps' *Phytovainetone* (bilberry).
Gerard's *Pilewort Compound* tablets (pilewort, senna, cranesbill, cascara).
Potter's *Pilewort* ointment, *Piletabs* (pilewort, agrimony, cascara, collinsonia).

Hair loss (Alopecia)

The cause of baldness is commonly genetic but can be due to general debility, stress or shock. Hair loss can be total, patchy, or confined to one or two relatively small circular patches. It is exacerbated by scaly conditions of the scalp such as dandruff, eczema and psoriasis. Genetic hair loss tends to be associated with age and hormonal change.

Certain drugs, especially if taken for prolonged periods, can cause toxicity and lead to hair loss.

When to seek professional help

It is important to assess any underlying problem of which the baldness is merely a symptom.

Diet and supplements

- See *What is a healthy diet?* on page 25.

Herbs

- **Rosemary** improves the blood flow to the head. It is also a nervous restorative. Externally it stimulates the hair follicles.

- **Nettles** are nutrious and tonifying and high in vitamins and minerals.

- **Burdock** is a blood cleanser, necessary where there is a build up of toxins and dandruff or an itchy and scaly scalp. An infusion can be made from equal parts of the herbs (grind the **burdock root**) using 1 tsp per cup to take 3 times a day. As a hair rinse, make three times the amount and use after each shampoo.

- **Rosemary oil**, 10 drops of essential oil in 10 ml of a base oil (such as olive) can be used to massage the scalp to stimulate the blood flow.

- Avoid harsh shampoos and chemical treatments to the hair and scalp, choosing a mild herbal product instead.

Available products

Cornucopia's *Rosemary and Lime* shampoo.
Potter's *Adiantine* (southernwood, bay oil, rosemary oil, witch hazel) and *Medicated Extract of Rosemary* (rosemary, rose geranium and bay oils).
Weleda's *Rosemary* shampoo.

Hay fever

This is an allergic reaction, most commonly to pollen, especially grass pollen, which causes sneezing, a runny nose, and red, streaming eyes. Sensitivity to tree resins and mould spores extends the symptom time to nearly the whole year. Hay fever is commonly a heredited predisposition associated with asthma and eczema. A food intolerance may be the trigger. Smoking and smoky atmospheres should be avoided. See *Allergies, Asthma, Catarrh*.

When to seek professional help

Allergic reactions can be very severe and the condition is often quite complex, so seek professional help.

Diet and supplements

- A food intolerance is most commonly due to dairy products or wheat (which is a grass), so this needs to be investigated.

- Onions, **garlic** and **horseradish** will help to lessen the allergic reaction. Vitamin C can be beneficial.

- See *What is a healthy diet?* on page 25.

Herbs

- **Elderflowers** and **eyebright** can help to bring relief as they are anti-inflammatory and anti-catarrhal. Use 1 to 2 tsp per cup to make an infusion and have this 2 to 3 times a day.

- **Nettles** have anti-allergic properties, as well as being cleansing and nourishing to the system. Have an infusion using 1 to 2 tsp per cup 2 to 3 times a day.

- **Golden seal**, infuse $\frac{1}{4}$ to $\frac{1}{2}$ tsp of the powdered herb and have 2 to 3 times a day to tone the mucous membranes (not to be used during pregnancy or with high blood pressure).

- **Ribwort** is a tonic, and healing to the mucous membranes.

- If the eyes are streaming and sore, use **eyebright** in an eyebath. Bathe the eyes as required.

- Alternatively, use **distilled witch hazel**, which can be chilled and applied with cotton wool pads placed over closed eyes or diluted in 3 to 5 parts boiled water and used to bathe the eyes.

- **Ephedra** is commonly suggested but this needs to be prescribed by a medical herbalist.

Headaches

Common causes of headaches include anxiety, allergy or food intolerance, constipation, high blood pressure, muscle tension, infections like influenza, sinusitis, spinal misalignment and stress. See *Allergies, Migraine*.

When to seek professional help

- If the headache comes after an accident or a blow to the head.

- If headaches are severe and not relieved by painkillers.

- If associated with any visual disturbance.

- If they have started recently and are becoming increasingly severe.

- Chiropractic or osteopathic techniques will help where there is some misalignment of the vertebrae in the neck. This is a common cause of headaches and particularly worth considering if you have had any accidents or have a history of backache.

- Massage of the head, neck and shoulders will relieve muscle tension, which is usually brought about by anxiety and stress.

Herbs

- Apply **lavender essential oil** neat to the temples, or use it diluted in a base vegetable oil (10 drops per 10 ml of base oil).

- Take **lavender tea** when required, using 1 to 2 tsp per cup for an infusion. This is a relaxant and tonic to the nervous system.

- **Rosemary** and **wood betony** are circulatory stimulants, especially to the head, and relaxing and restorative to the nervous system.

- **Skullcap** is also relaxant and restorative.

- **Marjoram** is warming and relaxing and can be used either as the essential oil or as a tea of the herb. Dosage for these is as for **lavender**.

Available products

Arkocaps' *Phytodreams* (Californian poppy).
Gerard's *Biophylin* tablets (valerian, skullcap, Jamaican dogwood, black cohosh).
Potter's *Anased Pain Relief* tablets (hops, Jamaican dogwood, wild lettuce, passiflora, pulsatilla), *Wood Betony and Skullcap Tablets No. 216.*

Hiatus hernia

This is a weakness of the cardiac sphincter, the valve which opens from the oesophagus into the stomach. This weakness leaves it prone to the regurgitation of acid from the stomach, which causes a burning sensation at the base of the breastbone above the stomach. Constipation, smoking, and being pregnant or overweight will aggravate the problem.

Antacids are best avoided, as with prolonged use, the stomach tends to increase acid output to compensate for the alkaline effect of the antacids. Many antacids are also aluminium-based, which apart from a possible association with senile dementia, can interfere with absorption from the digestive system. See also *Indigestion.*

When to seek professional help

Consider any spinal misalignment that might be contributing to the problem and consult an osteopath or chiropractor.

Exercise

Yoga exercises can help to strengthen and tone the abdomen.

Diet and supplements

- Lose weight if necessary.

- Try to eat little and often rather than eating large amounts at one sitting and allow time for eating.

- The Hay diet (see page 30) can prove effective.

- Eating late in the evening can cause severe discomfort, so try to allow several hours between eating and going to bed.

- Avoid eating acidic, fried, fatty and spicy foods.

- Coffee, tea and alcohol tend to increase stomach acidity, as does meat and excess milk consumption.

Herbs

- **Slippery elm**, powder or tablets, will soothe the digestive tract and protect it from the effects of the acid. It is probably best to experiment to see if it is most helpful to take it before, after or between meals.

- **Meadowsweet** reduces acidity and is soothing. Have 1 to 2 tsp per cup as an infusion 1 to 3 times a day.

- **Marshmallow root** is soothing and protective. Have a decoction of 1 tsp per cup 2 to 3 times a day.

- **Chamomile** is generally soothing and relaxing to the stomach. Have an infusion of 1 to 2 tsp per cup 1 to 3 times a day.

Available products

Gerard's *Papaya Plus* tablets (charcoal, papain, slippery elm, golden seal), *Golden Seal Compound* tablets (also marshmallow root, cranesbill, dandelion root).

High blood pressure (Hypertension)

High blood pressure is commonly a symptom of anxiety or stress but may be due to an allergy, kidney or glandular problem, drugs, obesity or pregnancy. Some people have a higher than normal blood pressure with no ill effect and no bodily imbalance. Lowering the blood pressure in such a case is likely to make the person feel unwell. See *Angina, Anxiety, Arteriosclerosis, Cholesterol, Stress.*

When to seek professional help

It is important to elicit the cause of the high blood pressure. If you are taking orthodox drugs and you wish to reduce these and also monitor your blood pressure, you will need to consult a medical herbalist.

Exercise

Exercise can aid the ability to relax and unwind where stress is a factor. The amount of exercise depends on the scale of the blood pressure. Yoga, relaxation, and breathing exercises can be particularly useful.

Diet and supplements

- Reduce your salt intake.

- Avoid caffeine, alcohol and cigarettes. See *What is a healthy diet?* on page 25, *Arteriosclerosis* and *Cholesterol*.

- Potassium is important for the healthy functioning of the heart. Orthodox diuretics and excess salt consumption deplete the body of this mineral. Good sources of potassium include bananas, grapes, oranges, potatoes and sunflower seeds. (Potassium needs to be restricted where there are kidney problems.)

Herbs

- **Hawthorn** berries and tops are a tonic to the heart and circulatory system. Have an infusion of 1 to 2 tsp per cup twice a day.

- **Cramp bark** will help to reduce blood pressure by relaxing the vessel walls and relieving general tension. Have a decoction of 1 tsp per cup 2 to 3 times a day.

- **Limeflowers** and **lemon balm** are relaxing, with an affinity for the heart and circulation. Have an infusion of 1 to 2 tsp per cup 2 to 3 times a day.

- **Dandelion leaf** will help to reduce blood pressure where there is also water retention. It is a diuretic and is very high in potassium. An infusion of 1 tsp per cup can be taken 2 to 3 times a day.

Available products

Gerard's *Motherwort Compound* tablets (also passionflower and limeflowers), *Hawthorn* tablets, *Cramp Bark* tablets.

Hypoglycaemia (Low blood sugar)

Symptoms include irritability, poor concentration, headaches, lethargy, weakness and a strong desire for something sweet. The cause is most commonly excessive consumption of refined carbohydrates, i.e. sugar, which causes blood sugar levels to soar shortly after consumption. Insulin is then released from the pancreas causing the blood sugar levels to drop dramatically and hunger to be initiated again. This disruption of the normally very stable blood sugar levels results in the pancreas becoming over-stressed and the delicate hormonal regulation of the body imbalanced. This can contribute to problems like premenstrual tension and thyroid conditions. See *Stress*.

When to seek professional help

- If the condition does not respond to dietary change.
- If it is associated with being very thirsty, an increased frequency in passing water and loss of weight.

Diet and supplements

- Try to eat small meals regularly, say every 2 to 3 hours.
- Avoid all sugar, alcohol, coffee, tea, chocolate, cocoa and cola drinks (caffeine has been shown to induce diabetes in children), and refined carbohydrates.
- High fibre foods and complex carbohydrates in the diet keep the blood sugar levels from rising dramatically, so have wholefoods like wholemeal bread, pasta, rice and potatoes.
- **Garlic**, leeks and onions, green beans, olive oil and artichokes are all beneficial in counteracting hypoglycaemia.
- Honey, dried fruit and concentrated fruit juices, are best restricted, especially if the condition is severe, until the condition is stabilised.
- If you are diabetic your fructose intake should not exceed 25 g per day, which is equivalent to about 150 g of sugar-free jam. See page 29 for alternatives to sugar, and *What is a healthy diet?* on page 25.

Herbs

- Bitter herbs help to counter hypoglycaemic attacks and restore the pancreatic function.
- Have a decoction of **dandelion root** using 1 to 2 tsp per cup 2 to 3 times a day.
- Have ½ a tsp of **gentian**, in tincture form, before each meal.
- **Swedish** or **Angostura bitters** could be taken instead.

Impotence

Likely causes are allergy, vitamin or mineral deficiency, drug side-effects, emotional or nervous involvement or a simple lack of desire.

Drugs or chemicals, prostate enlargement, nutritional deficiencies and psychological factors all need to be addressed. Many prescription drugs cause impotence. See *Anxiety, Depression, Prostate problems, Stress.*

When to seek professional help

Professional help is always advisable for this complex condition.

Diet and supplements

- It is usually best to remove direct stimulants, such as tea, coffee, chocolate, cocoa and cola drinks.

- See *What is a healthy diet?* on page 25.

Herbs

- **Saw palmetto** is a tonic to the male reproductive tract where there is general debility.

- **Damiana** is stimulating and enhancing, especially to the male reproductive system, where the problem is associated with a psychological or emotional element.

- Nervous restoratives such as oats and **rosemary** are useful for debilitated states and depression in both sexes.

- **Ginseng** is tonifying and strengthening and improves vitality in debilitated conditions.

Available products

Arkocaps' *Phytophrodisiac* (damiana).
Gerard's *Curzon* (damiana) tablets.
Potter's *Elixir of Damiana* and *Saw Palmetto* (also contains cornsilk).

Indigestion

Make sure that you are not eating too quickly. It is vital to make enough time to enjoy and digest meals. If you are rushed or anxious your body cannot cope with the digestion of food as well. Learning to relax will help, as tension creates poor blood supply to the digestive organs.

Antacids compound the situation as long-term suppression of stomach acid causes the body to over-compensate by producing increased amounts of acid necessary for the digestion of food. See *Anxiety, Bilious attack, Hiatus hernia, Stress.*

When to seek professional help

- If the pain is severe, if it radiates to your back, or if eating gives temporary relief, you may be suffering from a peptic ulcer.

- If it is accompanied by any change in bowel habit.

Diet and supplements

- Avoid specific foods that set off the indigestion, such as cheese, onion, cucumber or fried food.

- Consider the Hay diet (see page 30).

Herbs

- **Slippery elm** tablets are excellent for symptomatic relief of the discomfort. Take them before or after each meal depending on which works best for you.

- **Meadowsweet** will also settle the stomach and reduce excess acid production. **Caraway**, **dill** or **aniseed** will help to dispel the build-up of wind in the gut. **Peppermint** and **chamomile** are also excellent settlers. Use 1 to 2 tsp of herb or crushed seed per cup and take as required. A pinch of **ginger** can be added to any brew, and is particularly helpful where the digestive system has slowed with age.

Available products

Arkocaps' *Phytodigest* (artichoke).
Gerard's *Papaya Plus* tablets (slippery elm, golden seal, charcoal, papain), *Golden Seal Compound* tablets (also marshmallow root, cranesbill, dandelion root), *Ginger* tablets.
Potter's *Acidosis* (meadowsweet, charcoal, rhubarb, aniseed and caraway oils, cardamom and cinnamon), *Indian Brandee* (capsicum, ginger, rhubarb), *Indi-go No. 112A* (burnet greater, marshmallow root, meadowsweet, euonymus, hydrastis), *Appetiser Mixture and Indigestion Mixture* (meadowsweet, gentian, euonymus).

Influenza

Symptoms include fever, aching limbs, headache, coughing and nausea.
It is important to take 'flu seriously as it can be very debilitating. See
Catarrh, *Colds*, *Fever*, and *Convalescence* on page 13.

When to seek professional help

- If there is no improvement in 3 days or the temperature reaches 104°F
  (40°C).
- If it has been a severe bout of 'flu, see a medical herbalist for
  appropriate convalescent remedies.

Diet and supplements

- It is best to fast on fruit and vegetable juices as soon as the symptoms
  of 'flu become apparent.
- Beetroot boosts the immune system. It is available as juice, and can be
  mixed with apple or carrot juice to taste. Have a wineglassful as often
  as possible.
- Fresh **garlic** and **ginger** should be taken.

Herbs

Boneset, **echinacea**, **limeflowers** and **elderflower** teas should be drunk
freely. Use 1 to 2 tsp per cup.

Available products

Potter's *Influenza and Common Colds Mixture No. 86* (bayberry, boneset,
horehound, pinus canadensis, pleurisy root).

Insomnia

Disturbed nights tend to fall into two categories – either a difficulty in
getting off to sleep, or no problem with getting off to sleep, but a
tendency to wake after a few hours followed by difficulty getting back to
sleep. Many drugs cause sleeplessness due to irritation on the nervous
system. See *Anxiety*, *Depression*, *Stress*.

When to seek professional help

If you are relying on orthodox drugs such as sleeping tablets, or find you need to take the stronger sleep-inducing herbs on a regular basis, consult a medical herbalist.

Diet and supplements

- Avoid tea and coffee, especially after 6.00 p.m. You may need to stop them altogether as the effects can last many hours.

- Avoid chocolate and cola drinks which contain caffeine, and will keep you awake.

- A calcium and magnesium supplement, such as Dolomite, can prove beneficial, having a positive effect on the nervous system.

Herbs

- **Chamomile**, **lavender**, **lemon balm** and **limeflowers** are all relaxing plants so try these first. Have an infusion of 1 to 2 tsp per cup in the evening. Double the dose and brew twice to add to the bath.

- Add essential oils of **chamomile**, **lavender** and **lemon balm** to your bath – 10 drops in all.

- **Passionflower**, and **hops** and **valerian**, which are more specific sedatives, are stronger remedies to help induce sleep. Have an infusion of 1 to 2 tsp per cup in the evening. Avoid **hops** in depression.

Available products

Arkocaps' *Phytocarm* (passionflower), *Phytotranq* (valerian).
Gerard's *Biophylin* tablets (valerian, skullcap, Jamaican dogwood, black cohosh), *Passiflora* tablets, *99 Tablets* (hops, passionflower, valerian), *Valerian Compound* tablets (also hops).
Celestial Seasonings' *Sleepytime* and London Herb & Spice Co. *Golden Slumbers* teas are excellent.
Potter's *Newrelax* (hops, skullcap, valerian, vervain).

Kidney stones

Most kidney stones are composed of calcium oxalate, but some are composed of calcium phosphate, uric acid or cystine. Calcium stones are associated with high calcium levels in the blood. This can be due to excessive consumption of dairy foods or diseases like Cushing's syndrome or hyperparathyroidism, where the calcium metabolism is disrupted.

Urate stones are associated with excess secretion of uric acid, as occurs in gout.

Stones can be the result of kidney disease and can remain latent. There may be no pain apart from a dull ache in the loins.

Renal colic on the other hand is acutely painful and occurs when a stone is small enough to pass into the ureter. Pain is felt in the loins and radiates into the groin and is difficult to relieve. See *Cystitis, Gout*.

When to seek professional help

- If you have passed any blood or pus in your urine.

- If you are suffering from low back pain or fever.

- If you stop passing water.

Diet and supplements

- Reduce the amount of milk and milk products you eat (for alternatives see page 28).

- Avoid food rich in oxalates. These include spinach, rhubarb, strawberries, oranges, tomatoes, beetroot, peanuts, tea, coffee and chocolate.

- Make sure you are drinking enough, especially if you are physically very active. Try to have 1 or 2 litres of pure water a day. See the diet under *Gout*.

Herbs

- **Gravel root** helps the passage of kidney stones and is soothing and tonifying to the kidneys. A decoction of 1 tsp per cup can be taken 3 times a day.

- Marshmallow leaf helps to soothe the passage of the stones and **parsley piert** is soothing and restorative to the kidneys. 1 to 2 tsp per cup can be taken 3 times a day.

Liver disorders

The liver is the major detoxifying organ of the body. It plays a number of important roles in the vital functions of the body, including the regulation of blood sugar levels, the production of bile and the production of substances involved in blood clotting.

The liver can be disrupted after infections like hepatitis or any condition which has resulted in jaundice.

Excessive alcohol consumption will damage the liver and any allergic or toxic condition suggests strain on this organ. See *Bilious attack, Hypoglycaemia*, and *Convalescence* on page 13.

When to seek professional help

- If there is jaundice.
- If the condition is a result of an infection, alcohol abuse, or serious food or chemical poisoning.

Diet and supplements

- Alcohol, caffeine and fatty foods, especially saturated fats, need to be avoided, as these will only put extra strain on the liver.
- Artichokes, Jerusalem or globe, help to protect the liver.

Herbs

- **Dandelion root** and **milkthistle** are the best herbs to restore the liver. Have a decoction of 1 tsp per cup 3 times a day. It is worth maintaining this for at least 6 to 12 months.

Available products

Arkocaps' *Phytodigest* (artichoke).

ME (Myalgic encephalomyelitis)

Research seems to show that a virus is responsible for ME and the demonstrated reduced cellular respiration would support this theory.

The question that needs to be asked is why the virus has been able to become established. There is often a history of glandular fever, a stressful or very busy life-style or emotional turbulence. Other considerations include a low-grade infection such as a tooth abscess, heavy metal toxicity due to leakage or sensitivity to amalgam fillings in the teeth, or a food intolerance. Candida (Thrush) is sometimes implicated, but this is by no means inherent to the condition.

In practice, the causes are highly individual. It is a question of looking at the current problems, helping to support organs under stress or damaged by previous illness and improving the oxygen supply to the body's tissues. See *Anxiety, Candidiasis, Stress, How to survive modern living* on page 23 and the section about the immune system on page 12.

When to seek professional help

ME is best approached with a qualified practitioner. Apart from the wealth of diverse information available, which may, or may not be applicable to you, the severity of the condition is variable. Long-term sufferers take much longer to respond to treatment. Seek help as soon as you suspect ME might be your problem.

Exercise

- Breathing exercises are very useful (see page 31), also meditation.
- Rest is absolutely vital.

Diet and supplements

- See *What is a healthy diet?* on page 25.
- Check for any candida or food intolerances. Alcohol intolerance is common.
- Beetroot has been demonstrated to increase cell respiration and in practice has proved very helpful in ME. The suggested daily dose is up to 1 litre of juice per day.

Herbs

Herbs that stimulate the immune system, such as **echinacea**, which is most effective when taken regularly in small doses (10 drops of tincture or one tablet every 1 to 2 hours), are commonly indicated. **Echinacea** does not always suit everyone however. ME sufferers tend to be very sensitive to medication of any sort, dosages vary widely, and it is best to proceed with caution.

Menopausal problems

Symptoms can be quite diverse but often include hot flushes, anxiety, exhaustion, lack of sexual desire, vaginal discomfort, tension and depression. The sudden drop in oestrogen secretion at this time puts the other hormones out of balance. See also *Osteoporosis* and *Stress*.

When to seek professional help

- If the symptoms of the menopause are very severe, with depression, frequent hot flushes and night sweats causing distress and debilitation.

Diet and supplements

- Cut out tea, coffee, chocolate, cocoa and cola drinks, as the caffeine they contain is detrimental to the nervous system which is already strained and depleted.
- See *What is a healthy diet?* on page 25.

- **Evening primrose oil** is a good supplement to take.

Herbs

- **Yarrow**, **catmint** or **sage**, which have oestrogenic properties, can prove helpful for hot flushes.

- **Agnus castus** helps to balance the hormones and ½ to 1 tsp of the tincture should be taken first thing in the morning.

- **Ladies mantle** also helps to restore hormonal balance, as well as having a beneficial effect on the circulation.

- **Borage** helps to support the adrenal glands which take the strain of the hormonal changes occurring in the body.

- **Motherwort** is a useful relaxing tonic, particularly where there is accompanying anxiety and high blood pressure.

Available products

Gerard's *Agnacast* (agnus castus).

Migraine

Migraine is severe headache, often localised to one side of the head, associated with visual and digestive disturbance and nausea. It is commonly linked to anxiety and stress and the menstrual cycle in women. Spinal misalignment can be a contributory factor.

There appear to be two main types of migraine – those accompanied by constriction of the blood vessels in the head, relieved by placing hot packs on the head and those accompanied by dilation of the blood vessels, relieved by cold packs. See *Allergies, Anxiety, Bilious attack, Headaches, Liver disorders, Premenstrual tension, Stress*.

When to seek professional help

Due to the complexity of this condition, it is wise to seek thorough investigation and to consult a medical herbalist, especially where there is a strong dietary factor. Osteopathy or chiropractic manipulation is indicated to correct any misalignment of the neck or back. Cranial osteopathy is particularly effective in many cases of migraine.

Diet and supplements

- The most common food substances to trigger a migraine are tea, coffee, alcohol, chocolate, cheese and orange, so avoid these.

- Toxicity may be a factor, in which case a fast may be in order (see page 12).
- See also *What is a healthy diet?* on page 25.

Herbs

- Use the herbs suggested for *Headaches*.
- **Feverfew** dilates the blood vessels, is relaxant, anti-inflammatory and a bitter.
- Generally speaking, for migraines which are relieved by hot packs applied to the head, suitable remedies include **feverfew** and **rosemary**.
- For migraines relieved by cold packs, bitter remedies like **dandelion root** and **gentian** are suggested.

Available products

Arkocaps' *Phytodreams* (Californian poppy).
Gerard's *Biophylin* tablets (valerian, skullcap, Jamaican dogwood, black cohosh).
Potter's *Anased Pain Relief* tablets (hops, Jamaican dogwood, wild lettuce, passiflora, pulsatilla), *Wood Betony and Skullcap Tablets No. 216.*

Mouth ulcers

Mouth ulcers usually occur when you are run down, after an infection or stress. See *Gum disease, Stress.*

When to seek professional help

Consult your herbal practitioner if the condition is recurrent.

Diet and supplements

- Supplements of vitamin B complex and vitamin C are often beneficial.
- See *What is a healthy diet?* on page 25.

Herbs

Tormentil root is astringent, **myrrh** is astringent as well as antiseptic and healing and **marigold** is healing and astringent. A combination of equal parts of these herbs in tincture form make an effective mouthwash. Use 1 tsp in water at least twice a day.

Neuralgia

This is an acutely painful condition due to inflammation of a nerve sheath. It causes a stabbing or burning sensation along the path of the nerve and most commonly affects the face. It can also occur as a long-term problem after shingles or migraine. See *Shingles*.

When to seek professional help

- The condition might well require stronger herbs that need to be prescribed by a medical herbalist.
- Osteopathy or chiropractic is indicated to correct any misalignment of the neck and back, commonly the source of the problem.

Herbs

- A specific herb for this condition is **St John's wort**, which is anti-inflammatory and a nervous restorative.
- **Skullcap** is also restorative and a relaxant. Have an infusion of 1 to 2 tsp per cup 2 to 3 times a day.
- **St John's wort oil** can be applied over the affected area as often as required.
- **Peppermint essential oil** has analgesic properties and can be used neat on acutely painful neuralgia or diluted in the **St John's wort oil**.

Available products

Potter's *Sciatica Mixture No. 124A* (St John's wort, black cohosh, skullcap, juniper oil).

Osteoarthritis

This involves degeneration of the weight-bearing joints of the body, such as the hip, knee, ankle and spine. The cause is due to wear and tear on the joints which are under the most stress. This might be as a result of degeneration with age, or trauma inflicted through injury or occupation, for example sport, or even gardening. The erosion of the joint sets up an inflammatory response which exacerbates the condition. It is predominant in older women. See *Osteoporosis, Rheumatism and Arthritis, Menopausal problems*.

When to seek professional help

Osteopathic or chiropractic manipulation can be helpful by correcting any misalignment and correcting weight distribution.

Diet and supplements

- If necessary lose weight, as excess weight puts more stress on the joints.
- Refer to the dietary advice under *Osteoporosis* and *Rheumatism and Arthritis*.
- Dolomite (calcium and magnesium) can prove beneficial.

Herbs

- **Comfrey leaf** possesses remarkable healing properties which include promotion of growth of bone and cartilage tissue. 1 to 2 tsp per cup of the infusion should be taken 1 to 2 times a day.
- **Comfrey** might also be applied externally to the afflicted area as a compress or poultice (see page 20), or ointment. This is particularly beneficial with added **capsicum tincture**.
- **Horsetail** is extremely high in silica, a vital element for the healthy construction of connective tissue, and is an anti-inflammatory. 1 to 2 tsp per cup infused for 15 to 20 minutes should be taken 3 times a day.

Available products

Arkocaps'*Phytosilica* (bamboo).

Osteoporosis (Brittle bones)

This is a reduction in actual bone mass, causing susceptibility to fracture, typically the head of the femur in the hip joint and the spine.

The condition is most frequently found in post-menopausal, white women. The reduction in oestrogen with the menopause appears to reduce the ability to absorb calcium. There is also a dietary link and a healthy diet in early life is important in guarding against future problems.

Calcium is lost from the body in response to a high protein intake and large amounts of calcium are used during pregnancy and breast-feeding.

General lack of exercise and any immobilised joint can produce osteoporosis.

Prolonged steroid treatment (commonly prescribed, for example, to rheumatoid arthritis sufferers) and endocrine disorders, such as Cushing's syndrome, will also cause osteoporosis. See *Menopausal problems, Osteoarthritis*.

When to seek professional help

It is sensible to seek sound individual guidance on diet and supplements.

Action

Stop smoking and re-evaluate the use of steroids as these contribute to osteoporosis, as does the contraceptive pill.

Diet and supplements

- Reduce the amount of animal protein, especially meat, in your diet.

- Do not rely on dairy produce as your main source of calcium.

- Rich sources of calcium include sesame seeds, sunflower seeds, almonds, hazelnuts (made into spreads and nut butters, available from health foods shops), dark-green, leafy vegetables, kelp and canned fish such as sardines (in their own oil).

- Take a tablespoon of apple cider vinegar in water with honey before meals, to promote the absorption of calcium from the digestive tract.

- Most calcium is lost at night, so it is sensible to eat and drink calcium-rich products in the evening.

- Dolomite (calcium and magnesium) is an excellent supplement. See *What is a healthy diet?* on page 25.

Herbs

- **Kelp** is highly nutritive. It is also a gentle stimulant and a tonic to the metabolism, beneficial where there is imbalance in the glandular system and in arthritic conditions. It is available widely in tablet form.

- **Borage** and **natural liquorice root** might be taken for their restorative action on the adrenal glands.

Painful periods (Dysmenorrhoea)

The pain associated with a menstrual period can begin a day or more before the flow starts, or can accompany the flow and diminish after the first day or two. The first picture suggests congestion in the pelvis, the second very tense or dysfunctioning uterine muscles.

The severe cramping pain can be debilitating, causing nausea and fainting, and be associated with heavy blood loss and diarrhoea. The pain commonly radiates down the legs.

Assess the general circulation in the body and try to avoid constipation, particularly leading up to the period. See *Premenstrual tension, Constipation, Circulatory problems.*

When to seek professional help

- If there is no improvement within three months.
- If the pain is accompanied by very heavy menstrual flow.

Exercise

- Daily exercise the rest of the month can improve the situation, helping to stimulate the circulation and relieve congestion. Walking, swimming, running, cycling, riding and yoga are all beneficial.
- Warm baths and hot water bottles can bring symptomatic relief. Alternating hot and cold showers over the abdomen and lower back throughout the month stimulates the circulation and relieves congestion.

Herbs

- **Black haw** or **cramp bark** are effective in relieving painful cramping and have a general relaxing effect. They also help to relieve a very heavy period.
- **Blue cohosh** and **black cohosh** are also antispasmodic and relax the uterus. They also have a normalising action on the reproductive system.
- **Valerian** could also be used as a muscle relaxant. All these herbs need to be made up as decoctions, use 1 to 2 tsp per cup, apart from **black cohosh** for which the dose is $\frac{1}{2}$ tsp per cup.

Palpitations

These can be described as a 'fluttering heart' and can be quite disturbing. They are, however, simply an awareness of the heart beating. Most commonly attributed to nervous tension, consumption of caffeine, or occasioned by exercise or a feverish illness, they can be accompanied by shortness of breath. They are most usually a benign symptom of nervous over-stimulation to the heart. See *Anxiety and Stress.*

When to seek professional help

If the condition is not relieved by the suggested measures and relaxing herbs.

Diet

Cut all caffeine out of your diet. This includes coffee, tea, chocolate and cola drinks. These will be constantly stressing your nervous system and stimulating adrenalin secretion, which in turn stimulates the heart. For alternatives see page 29.

Herbs

Lemon balm, **limeflowers** or **motherwort** might be taken. All are relaxing herbs with an affinity for the heart and circulation. Make an infusion of 1 to 2 tsp per cup 2 to 3 times a day.

Premenstrual tension (PMT)

Symptoms include weight gain, tender breasts, headaches, irritability, tearfulness, sugar craving, inability to sleep, fatigue, depression and lowered resistance to infection. See *Anxiety, Hypoglycaemia, Stress, Water retention*.

When to seek professional help

Balancing the hormones can be complex, and there is often more to the picture. If the situation shows no signs of improvement within three months see a qualified herbalist. There is a wealth of herbs for the reproductive and hormonal system but these need to be tailored to the individual.

Exercise

Regular exercise throughout the month can help considerably. This might be walking, running, riding, dancing, yoga or similar. This will not only help to reduce stress levels but balance the hormones.

Diet and supplements

- Hypoglycaemia, otherwise known as *sugar craving*, is notorious before a period in sufferers of premenstrual tension, but this is controllable through diet and eating regular meals (see *Hypoglycaemia*).
- See *What is a healthy diet?* on page 25.
- Supplements of magnesium, zinc and B complex can be taken if necessary.

- **Evening primrose oil** supplies essential fatty acids.

Herbs

- **Agnus-castus** is a hormone balancer. It acts on the pituitary gland, the master gland governing the body, and regulates hormone function. If using the tea, crush 1 tsp of the seeds and infuse for 10 minutes. Drink this first thing in the morning, when the pituitary is most active. The tincture could be taken instead, ½ to 1 tsp in the mornings. It is also available in tablet form. If you have a regular cycle, take the **agnus-castus** for the second half of your cycle only, from ovulation to menstruation (approximately day 14 to day 28). If your cycle is irregular, or the symptoms are very severe, take it for the whole month. This needs to be taken for at least three months.

- **Borage** can be taken as an infusion of 1 to 2 tsp per cup 2 to 3 times a day, as a tonic and restorative.

Available products

Gerard's *Agnacast* (agnus-castus).

Prostate problems

The early signs are a weakened flow of urine leading to difficulty starting and stopping the flow. Symptoms include urgency, incontinence, night-time visits to the toilet and dribbling. The enlargement of this gland is associated with decreased sexual activity following a change in hormone levels. It is an extremely common condition of ageing in men.

When to seek professional help

- If urination suddenly becomes difficult or painful.
- If blood is visible in urine or semen.

Exercise

- Pelvic floor exercises are beneficial.
- Another precaution is to maintain an active sexual life and general exercise.

Diet and supplements

- Eating sunflower and, especially, pumpkin seeds daily will supply nutrients to maintain a healthy prostate.

- When the gland has become enlarged, and definitely if it is inflamed, it is wise to become vegetarian for at least three months, or until all signs of the inflammation have gone.

Herbs

- In the early stages of prostate enlargement, or even as a precautionary measure, drink **nettle tea**, 1 to 2 tsp per cup, once or twice a day.

- **Saw palmetto** is a tonic to the male reproductive system, particularly the prostate. It is also anti-infective. Take a decoction of ½ to 1 tsp of the berries 2 to 3 times a day.

- **Hydrangea** (not the garden variety) **root** is specific when the prostate is inflamed.

- When inflamed, soothing and anti-infective measures need to be taken. See *Cystitis*.

Available products

Potter's *Protat* tablets (cornsilk, kava).

Psoriasis

This skin condition is notoriously difficult to treat. It usually appears as well-defined, reddened, circular patches on the body or face, covered with a silvery-white, scaly layer which flakes off. Sometimes lesions become pustular. Severe cases need expert diagnosis.

Psoriasis can affect the scalp, the nails (which become pitted) and inside the ears. It can become intensely itchy and there is a tendency for it to improve and then regress. It is an autoimmune disease (see page 12), causing inflammation and over-proliferation of skin cells. The condition can be quite severe and be associated with arthritis. It is common in young adults.

Familial disposition, the build-up of toxins, including the deposition of metals like aluminium, and any areas of weakness, such as the liver, lungs, kidneys or acute or chronic illness that might be stressing the system need to be assessed. Anxiety and stress are often factors. See *Allergies*, *Anxiety*, *Stress*.

When to seek professional help

Psoriasis is a very complex disease and it is worth seeking a professional opinion. Treatment needs to be maintained long-term which can be discouraging. It is necessary to isolate any food intolerances, environmental factors and organ weaknesses.

Diet and supplements

- Avoid caffeine-containing foods, such as coffee, tea, chocolate and soft drinks.

- Restrict the consumption of pig meat, plaice, mackerel, tuna, shellfish, convenience food, sugar and dairy products.

- Cold-pressed oils should be included generously in the diet.

- Take **evening primrose oil**, up to 3 g per day.

Herbs

- **Cleavers** is a lymphatic cleanser and helps promote the excretion of toxic products from the body. Have an infusion of 2 to 3 tsp per cup 3 to 4 times a day.

- **Dandelion root** is a tonic and decongestant to the liver, stimulating excretion of waste products. Take this as a decoction or grind the roasted root and make as filter coffee, using 1 to 2 tsp per cup twice a day.

- **Burdock root** is particularly effective at cleansing the tissues of toxic waste and is indicated where metals have accumulated in the body. This may be taken in the same way as **dandelion root**, and at the same time, but care must be taken with the dosage as it can have a very powerful effect and precipitate a crisis in severely toxic conditions. It is best to start cautiously, then gradually increase the dose. Use $\frac{1}{2}$ to 1 tsp 2 to 3 times a day.

- **Burdock** may also be applied externally as a compress or poultice.

- **Yellow dock root** can be used as an alternative or in combination with **burdock** (proceed cautiously).

- Any of the above might be used in external applications, as can cold-pressed oils and **evening primrose oil**.

- **Calendula** or **chamomile** ointment can be helpful, also **essential oil of tagetes** diluted 1 drop per ml of ointment or oil.

Available products

Gerard's *Blue Flag Root Compound* tablets (blue flag, burdock, sarsaparilla). Potter's *Skin Eruptions Mixture No. 83* (blue flag, burdock, yellow dock, sarsaparilla, cascara, buchu).

Rheumatism and arthritis

This covers a wide range of conditions which involve the inflammation of joints and muscles. The picture commonly involves the accumulation of toxins in the tissues, digestive problems, constipation, poor circulation, kidney weakness, food intolerances and psychological factors.

The aim of treatment is to stimulate elimination and circulation, relieve the inflammation and treat underlying factors like stress. See *Allergies, Gout, Neuralgia, Osteoarthritis, Osteoporosis, Stress.*

When to seek professional help

Due to the complex nature and variations in severity of this condition, it is advisable to consult a practitioner to devise the best treatment plan for you.

Exercise

- This helps to maintain mobility and blood supply to the joints. Swimming, yoga and T'ai chi or just simple stretch exercises are suitable.

- With a flare up of arthritic symptoms, exercise should be kept to an absolute minimum.

- Relaxation, visualisation and breathing exercises should be incorporated into your daily life.

Diet and supplements

- See *What is a healthy diet?* on page 25.

- Avoid coffee, tea, red meat (pork, beef, lamb), sugar, refined and processed foods, food additives, vinegar (except apple cider vinegar) and pickles, alcohol, oranges and yeast concentrates like Bovril and Marmite.

- Dairy products should be kept to a minimum and avoided completely if there is any sensitivity to milk (see page 28).

- Wheat consumption should also be curtailed and should be investigated for any sensitivity, as it is a very common allergen.

- The advice on citrus fruits is contradictory – although oranges should be avoided, grapefruit and lemons can be extremely effective in relieving arthritis. Although they are acid to eat, once metabolised by the body they become alkaline, so neutralising the acidity produced by arthritic conditions. The usefulness of these fruits is dependent upon the type of arthritis – citrus fruits being cooling where the condition is accompanied by hot and swollen joints.

- Avoid rhubarb, beetroot, tomatoes, spinach, strawberries and oranges which are all high in oxalic acid which tends to aggravate arthritic joints.

- Red cherries actively dissolve uric acid crystals and can be eaten freely when in season.

- Apple cider vinegar with a little honey, up to 1 tbsp 3 times a day, can be remarkably effective. Apart from making the system alkaline, it helps dispel toxins from the system and supplies essential minerals.

- The Hay diet (see page 30) can prove very beneficial.

- Detoxification might be required, see page 11 on elimination and fasting.

- Fish oils, for example cod liver oil, which is readily available as a liquid or in capsules from health food shops and chemists, and **evening primrose** oil can be indispensable.

- If anaemia is associated with the condition, Floradix iron supplement is an excellent, readily absorbed source of iron and the B vitamins and a general tonic.

Herbs

- **Celery seeds** stimulate the secretion of uric acid via the kidneys. Crush and infuse 1 to 2 tsp and take 3 times a day.

- **Birch** is diuretic and anti-inflammatory and helps support the kidneys.

- **Meadowsweet** and **willow bark** are both anti-inflammatory and help to deal with the pain and flush uric acid out of the system.

- The addition of a circulatory stimulant, such as **prickly ash**, and a potent tissue cleanser, such as **burdock**, increases the overall effect.

- Take herbs to support the liver, like **dandelion root**.

- **Boneset** might be employed where the condition is aggravated by damp or constipation.

- **Black cohosh** is particularly useful in neuralgias and muscular pain.

- **Bogbean** is effective where the condition is associated with constipation or poor digestion.

- Other herbs that can be considered include **devil's claw**, **guaiacum**, **wintergreen** and **white poplar**.

- Treat externally with essential oils of **juniper**, **rosemary** and **wintergreen**, or **marjoram**.

- Place poultices (see page 20) of $\frac{1}{2}$ tsp of **cayenne**, 1 to 2 tsp fresh **horseradish** or 1 tsp of **mustard** powder per tbsp of **slippery elm**

powder or mashed potato or porridge over the affected joints to stimulate the blood supply to the area. Take care not to leave these on too long, as they can cause blistering. Start cautiously with 5 to 10 minutes, gradually increasing the length of time.

- Where the joint is very hot and swollen, use essential oils of **juniper**, **lavender** and **peppermint** in the poultice or in a linament.

- Epsom salt baths are useful for drawing out body toxins. Put $\frac{1}{2}$ kg in a hot bath and soak in it for 20 minutes. Do this once a week.

- **Caution.** Epsom salt baths are not advisable for people with high/low blood pressure or heart conditions.

Available products

Potter's *Tabritis* (elderflowers, prickly ash, yarrow, burdock, cleavers, poplar bark, uva ursi), *Rheumatic Pain Tablets* (bogbean, yarrow, burdock, guaiacum, nutmeg), *Rheumatism Tablet No. 31* (rhubarb, guaiacum, blue flag, uva ursi), *Rheumatic Pain Mixture No. 92* (black and blue cohosh, juniper, burdock, cascara), *Rheumatism Mixture No. 92A* (willow, black and blue cohosh, burdock, yarrow). *Nine Rubbing Oils.*
Gerard's *Ligvites* and *Celery* tablets, *Dragon Balm* ointment.

Shingles

This is characterised by painful blisters which appear at the nerve endings, usually on one side of the face or body. It is caused by the same virus that causes chicken pox and can lie dormant to reappear when you become run down. There should be long- and short-term strategies employed to overcome the virus. Short-term, the virus needs to be quelled and damage repaired in order that no long term nerve damage is caused. See *Stress*, *Neuralgia* and *Convalescence* on page 13.

Diet and supplements

- Avoid tea, coffee, cola drinks, cocoa and chocolate.

- Include cold-pressed oils, such as safflower, sunflower and linseed.

- Beetroot (1 tumblerful to 1 litre of the juice per day), **garlic** and **evening primrose** are all beneficial.

When to seek professional help

If the nerve supplying the eye is affected, consult your doctor immediately.

Herbs

- Take **echinacea** as tea or tablets every hour initially.

- Use **St John's wort oil** as it is not only anti-inflammatory but helps to repair the damaged nerve. Apply it 3 times a day, and take the tea of the same herb internally.

- **Essential oil of peppermint** is pain-killing and can be added to **St John's wort oil** or any cold-pressed oil at the rate of 1 to 2 drops of essential oil per 1 ml of base oil. **Lavender essential oil** could be used too.

Sinusitis

Congestion of the sinuses with mucus results in inflammation of the tissues and causes pain. The sinuses need to be cleared of mucus and the membranes healed. See *Catarrh*.

When to seek professional help

- If the condition does not respond to the suggestions in this book.

- If the condition is recurrent.

Diet and supplements

Avoid dairy products completely during the acute stage and for a month after, to allow healing of the mucous membranes.

Action

Apply alternately hot and cold flannels to the face. This stimulates blood flow and will reduce the congestion.

Herbs

- **Eyebright** or **elderflower tea** with two slices of **ginger** added will start to clear the congested nasal passages.

- Apply the excellent mix of tinctures consisting of equal parts of **lobelia**, **myrica**, **hydrastis**, **capsicum** and **myrrh**. This must only be used externally and can be obtained from a herbalist.

- Inhalations using a strong infusion of **chamomile tea** can bring relief. Essential oils of **eucalyptus** and **lavender** can be added.

Sore throat (and Laryngitis)

Inflammation of the throat, which if it involves the voice box, the larynx, causes hoarseness or loss of voice and is called *laryngitis*. Recurrent sore throats suggest a wider problem, possibly involving a systemic disorder or lowered immune system, or food intolerance. See *Allergies, Catarrh, Colds, Coughs, Influenza*.

When to seek professional help

- Any case of hoarseness which goes on for more than a few weeks, or gradually worsens.
- Recurrent sore throats.
- Any throat infection needs competent and speedy help.

Action

If the throat is a susceptible area, singing can help to strengthen it and also release tension.

Diet and supplements

- Avoid all dairy products.
- Take 1 g of vitamin C a day to boost the immune system and healing.

Herbs

- **Red sage** (to be avoided during pregnancy) and **thyme** are both antiseptic and astringent. Infuse 2 to 3 tsp per cup and gargle with this while still warm. **Rosemary** or **eucalyptus** might also be used, and a few grains of **cayenne** added to the gargle will add to the effect.
- **Myrrh** or **balm of gilead**, are also beneficial as they are antiseptic, astringent and healing. Due to their resinous nature, take them as tinctures. Add ½ tsp to the above infusion or warm water and gargle. The gargle may be repeated as often as every couple of hours, reducing to once or twice a day until the symptoms have cleared.
- Essential oils of **thyme**, **tea tree** and **myrrh** might be used in a gargle. A total of 3 drops should be used per cup of infusion or simply in warm water.
- Mucilagenous herbs to soothe a very inflamed throat include **marshmallow root**, and **liquorice root**. Any of these might be made up as a decoction using 1 to 2 tsp per cup and sipped at regular intervals.
- **Hibiscus tea** can make a very soothing drink. Honey might be added to any of these.

- Compresses of the above herbs can also be applied externally.
- Gargles should not be swallowed unless instructed to do so by a practitioner.

Available products

Potter's *Genuine Composition Essence* (capsicum, ginger and oak bark), *Life Drops* (capsicum and elderflowers with peppermint oil) and *Peerless Composition Essence* (oak bark, hemlock spruce, poplar bark, prickly ash bark and bayberry bark in syrup with capsicum oil).
Weleda's *Mouthwash & Gargle*.

Stress

Stress is a normal part of a balanced life. However, when we are overwhelmed by stress we are constantly producing adrenaline, which, over prolonged periods, prevents correct digestion and body maintenance. See *Anxiety, Depression, Insomnia* and *How to survive modern living* on page 23.

Exercise

- Make sure you get sufficient exercise, as this uses up the adrenaline.
- Take time to do yoga, swimming or breathing exercises, as these turn off the adrenaline production. Breathing exercises can become a continuous part of life, hence maintaining a relaxed state. This in turn will help you rest and sleep.

Diet and supplements

- It is important not to neglect your diet because of lack of time. See *What is a healthy diet?* on page 23.
- Foods rich in B vitamins (yeast extract, brewer's yeast) help to nourish a stressed nervous system.
- Oatmeal or groats (more nutritious than rolled oats) as porridge or in a muesli, help to feed the nervous system.
- Raw, cold-pressed oils (sunflower, safflower, olive) and/or **evening primrose** oil capsules are also important for the nutrition of the nervous system.
- Caffeine intake should be strictly curtailed, see page 29.

Herbs

- **Skullcap**, **St John's wort** and **vervain** are all relaxing with a restorative and tonic effect on the nervous system. Infuse 1 to 2 tsp per cup 2 to 3 times a day.

- **Borage** helps to support the adrenal glands.

Available products

Potter's *Trucalm Elixir* (oats, passionflower, vervain, skullcap), *Stresses and Strains Herb* (hops, skullcap, valerian, vervain, wood betony).

Thrush

This vaginal discharge resembles cottage cheese in colour and consistency. It itches intensely and can become very sore.

The yeast-like fungus responsible for thrush is also known as *candida albicans*, and commonly proliferates when taking the Pill, after antibiotics, or during pregnancy, when there is a lack of oestrogen, which normally maintains the bacteria responsible for keeping the yeast cells in check. The acid–alkali balance of the vagina becomes sweeter and is an ideal habitat for the thrush to grow in.

Thrush can be passed to the baby as it goes through the vagina during birth or to a woman's sexual partner. See also *Candidiasis*.

When to seek professional help

- If the discharge has an odour, or becomes coloured, another organism may be present, in which case ask your doctor about having a swab taken.

Diet and supplements

- Cutting out sugar is vital. This includes all foods containing sugar and alcohol (which is basically fermented sugar).

- If the problem is recurrent, turn to the entry for *Candidiasis*.

- Superdophilus, Acidophilus or Probion as tablets, capsules or powder can be taken.

- Eat live, natural yoghurt.

- Cider vinegar can be diluted 1 tbs (15 ml) per pint (500 ml) and used to wash the vagina with, or added to the bath.

- Probion pessaries or live yoghurt (via a tampon or its applicator or a syringe without the needle) can be inserted into the vagina.

- Use towels as opposed to tampons during your period.

Herbs

- **Tea tree oil** has antifungal properties and is available in pessaries which can be inserted into the vagina.

- Add 2 to 3 drops each of **tea tree**, **lavender** and **myrrh essential oil** or 6 drops of one to a bidet or equivalent and wash the affected area. Alternatively, dilute the essential oil in 20 ml of olive oil and apply it to the area with cotton wool.

- **Lavender**, **marigold**, **rosemary**, **thyme** and **white deadnettle tea** ($\frac{1}{2}$ tsp of each or 3 tsp of one, per cup), can be used as a wash for the area or as a douche as often as required.

- **Calendula** (marigold) cream or ointment could be used, as it has antifungal properties. The essential oils mentioned above could be added to this, at 1 drop per 10 ml of cream, or diluted in 20 ml of olive oil and applied, using cotton wool.

- Take **echinacea** to boost the immune system. Make a decoction of 1 tsp per cup and drink 1 to 3 times a day. This can also be used to wash the area.

- **Golden seal** (do not use during pregnancy) is a tonic to the mucous membranes and can be used as a douche, or taken as a tea. Make a decoction of $\frac{1}{2}$ tsp per cup and take 2 to 3 times a day as a tea.

Available products

Arkocaps' *Phytokold* (echinacea).
Gerard's *Echinacea, Echinacea and Garlic* tablets.
House of Mistry's *Tea tree pessaries*.
Potter's *Antifect* (echinacea and garlic).

Tinnitus

Ringing in the ears can be caused by catarrh, drugs, nerve damage or poor circulation. Herbal treatment revolves around using herbs that support the nervous system and circulation, See *Anxiety, Arteriosclerosis, Circulatory problems* and *Stress*.

Diet and supplements

- Stop drinking tea, coffee, cola drinks and cocoa.

- Cold-pressed oils should be consumed.

- Take **oil of evening primrose** or **linseed** throughout treatment.

When to seek professional help

- Always see a qualified practitioner for a correct diagnosis.
- If accompanied by dizziness or hearing loss.
- If drug reduction is involved.

Herbs

- **Skullcap** and **St John's wort** are the best herbs, used alongside **wood betony** and the **ginkgo**, which stimulate blood flow to the head.
- Another plant to consider is **lesser periwinkle**.

Available products

Arkopharma's *Phytomemo* (maiden hair tree).
Gerard's *Ginkgo*.

Varicose veins

Hereditary factors often play a part in the tendency to varicose veins.
   They commonly appear during pregnancy, particularly after the first baby.
   With the effects of gravity there is a tendency for the blood to pool in the lower part of the body, stretching the veins. The legs can ache and feel heavy and the veins can irritate. Standing will aggravate symptoms.
   Constipation, water retention and excessive weight gain can all contribute to the problem. Long-term treatment is needed to restore tone. See *Haemorrhoids* (Piles), *Circulatory problems*.

When to seek professional help

- If the leg/s or vein becomes hot, tender, swollen or infected.
- If the vein becomes ulcerated.

Exercise

- Walking regularly, and briskly, improves the circulation and helps to pump the blood from the legs back to the heart.
- Avoid standing for long periods of time. If you have to stand, contract your calves, move your feet and toes, and go up on tiptoes periodically. Support tights would be of benefit here.

- Avoid crossing your legs.
- Put your feet up as much or as regularly as possible.
- Rinsing your legs down with cold water can help to astringe the veins.
- Use ice packs to relieve inflamed and aching veins.

Diet and supplements

- Eat foods rich in vitamin C (fruit and vegetables) and vitamin E (wheatgerm and sunflower seeds) should be eaten.
- Buckwheat is high in rutin, and will help to strengthen blood vessel walls and promote healing. Rutin is available as a tea or in tablets.
- Blue and black fruit such as plums, blackberries, blueberries, dark cherries and blackcurrants provide bioflavonoids which are important for the integrity of the blood vessel walls.

Herbs

- **Witch hazel bark**, **bistort** and **horsechestnut** will astringe and tone the veins. Make a decoction using 2 tsp of the mixture per cup. Apply cold (or frozen into ice-cubes). These herbs, in tincture form, could be made up into a cream.
- **Calendula** and **comfrey** are healing and anti-inflammatory. These are best used in the form of a cream or ointment. Apply creams with sweeping upward strokes.

Available products

Arkocaps' *Phytovainetone* (bilberry), *Phytovarix Massage Gel for Tired Legs* (red vine, butcher's broom, witch hazel, horsechestnut, menthol, essential oils of cypress, lavender).
Potter's *Varicose Ointment*.

Warts and verrucas

These tend to appear when the body's immune system is low. They are caused by a virus which produces an excess of what can be unsightly skin growth. They are slightly contagious.

It is worth checking internal factors such as diet, immunological health and circulation.

When to seek professional help

- If you suspect you have genital warts.

Herbs

- The most effective external applications are the fresh, milky sap from the stem of the **dandelion** or the yellow sap from the stem of **greater celandine**.

- Internally, tincture of **thuja** is particularly effective with verrucas. This can be obtained from a medical herbalist. Take 10 drops in a little water twice a day.

Water retention (Oedema)

This is most commonly characterised by swelling of the fingers, ankles or feet, which is aggravated by standing and hot weather, and is worse at the end of the day. It is more likely to occur in women, where it is often associated with the menstrual cycle or pregnancy.

The cause may lie with the heart and circulation, poor kidney function, allergy or toxic overload in the body.

It is important to assess any medication that is being taken, including orthodox diuretics, which, if taken long-term, can compound the problem. See *High blood pressure*.

When to seek professional help

- It is important to establish the cause of the water retention.

- In pregnancy, when oedema is associated with high blood pressure, protein in the urine and headaches, toxaemia is likely and **urgent** help is required.

- If the heart needs support or you are taking any other medication, you should consult a medical hebalist.

Diet and supplements

Salt intake should be minimised. Salt is present in processed, packet and canned foods, pickles, sauces, butter, smoked foods, cheese, nuts, dried meats and fish, sausages, bacon and cured meats.

Herbs

- **Celery seeds** (not during pregnancy) are diuretic and flush any toxic build-up of uric acid out of the system. An infusion of 1 tsp of the freshly crushed seeds can be taken 2 to 3 times a day.

- **Cleavers** can be used similarly where there is toxic congestion, to clear the lymphatic tissue. An infusion of 1 to 2 tsp per cup can be taken 2 to 3 times a day.

- **Dandelion** herb can be used as a diuretic when the condition is uncomfortable. This herb is extremely high in potassium, unlike orthodox diuretics which deplete the body of this important mineral. An infusion of 1 to 2 tsp per cup can be taken 1 to 3 times a day.

- **Horsetail** could be used as an alternative diuretic, especially with hormonal problems.

- **Parsley piert** is a kidney restorative and will help to improve kidney function, as well as support the kidneys while the body is being flushed of toxins. Have an infusion of 1 to 2 tsp per cup 2 to 3 times a day.

Available products

Gerard's *Celery* tablets, *Waterlex* tablets (dandelion, horsetail, uva ursi). Potter's *Watershed Mixture No. 110* (wild carrot, pellitory, juniper, cleavers, buchu).

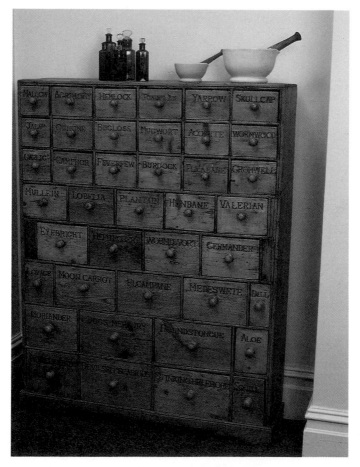

A set of Victorian spice drawers used for herbs

7

THE KITCHEN PHARMACY

Allspice (pimento)
- Aromatic, stimulant
- Useful for flatulent indigestion

Angelica
- A warming digestive
- Especially helpful for stomach

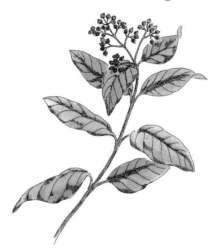

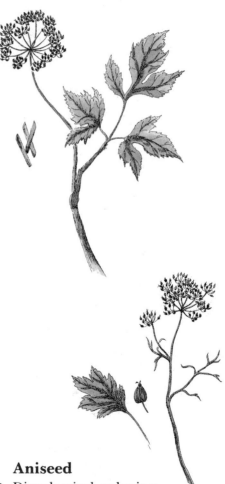

Almonds
- Good source of calcium and useful general tonic
- Especially soothing to lungs, genito urinary system

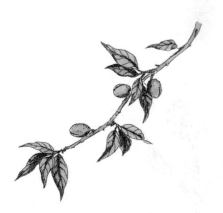

Aniseed
- Dispels wind, relaxing, antiseptic expectorant
- Use for dry coughs, asthma, whooping cough, infantile catarrh, flatulence, colic

Apples

- Rich in vitamins, digestive enzymes, essential acids, and minerals
- Aid digestion and prevent liver disturbance, neutralise acidity in the stomach and tissues
- Ease constipation as contain pectin, an aperient and cleanser of noxious substances from the body's tissues
- A tooth cleaner and gum strengthener
- Apple juice recommended for dissolving gallstones and kidney stones. Drink 1 to 2 litres per day
- A glass of apple cider taken regularly will prevent kidney stones forming
- Apple cider vinegar only vinegar which does not increase acidity of the blood. An excellent tissue cleanser with fine tradition of use as arthritis cure

Apricots

- High in iron, so used with anaemia

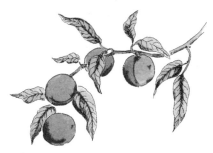

Arrowroot

- Nourishing, easily digested
- Particularly good for digestive upsets

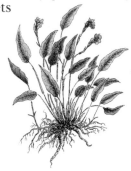

Artichoke, globe and Jerusalem

- Stimulate liver cell regeneration
- Tonic to kidneys
- Soothe and gently stimulate intestines
- Cholesterol reducing properties
- Contain insulin-like substances, so helpful in diabetes

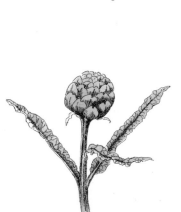

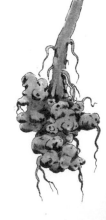

Asparagus

- Diuretic, laxative
- Kidney cleanser
- Contains amino acid essential for growth, division, regeneration of cells
- Juice helps break up oxalic acid and crystals in kidneys, so useful in kidney stones, rheumatism, arthritis
- A general tonic

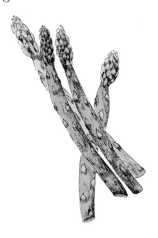

Avocado

- Rich source of protein and a rare digestible oil
- Rich in potassium, folic acid, vitamin A

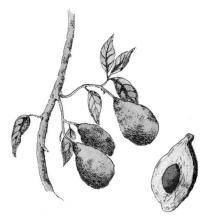

Banana

- High in potassium, so aids some cases of high blood pressure
- Mucus forming, however, so to be avoided in catarrhal conditions

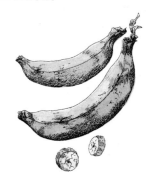

Barley

- For febrile conditions and catarrhal conditions of respiratory and urinary systems
- Barley water eases cystitis

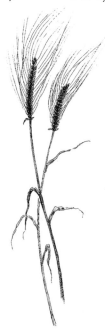

Basil

- Brings mental acuity, while relaxing, so aiding memory
- Relieves flatulence, indigestion, colds, headaches
- Plant kept in the house said to purify the space (certainly discourages flies)

Beetroot

- Immune stimulant and vitality enhancer
- Used with great benefit for cancer, leukaemia, ME patients
- Known as blood builder for centuries as high in iron

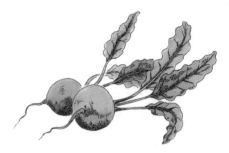

Black- and redcurrants

- Useful sources of vitamin C
- Astringe and heal sore throats
- Diuretic
- Aid toning of varicose veins and capillaries, reducing bruising

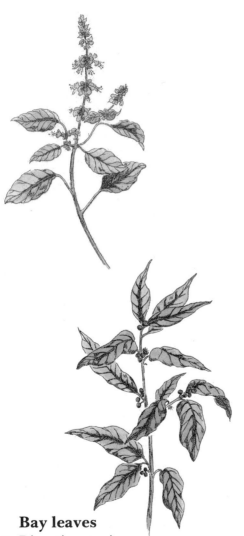

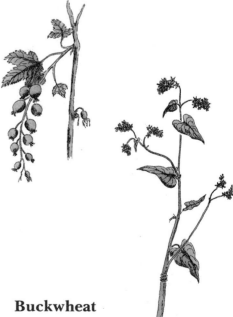

Bay leaves

- Digestive, tonic
- Ease bloating after meals
- Diuretic
- Dry the mucus of colds, bronchitis

Buckwheat

- Contains rutin so will aid toning of varicose veins and capillaries, reducing bruising

Cabbage

- Poultices excellent for inflamed joints caused by rheumatism, overwork
- Poultices greatly aid mastitis as cooling and draining
- Drink cabbage juice for ulcers, indigestion, cystitis

Carrots

- Produce vitamin A, so reputation for improving eyesight not without grounds
- Anti-inflammatory and stabilising to bowel function so used in irritable bowel, especially as fresh juice

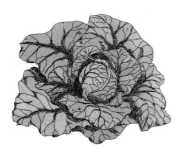

Caraway

- Digestive aid
- Reduces wind in intestines
- A general tonic

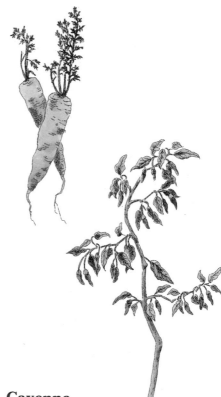

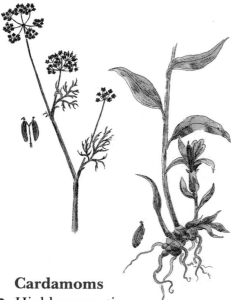

Cardamoms

- Highly aromatic
- Relieve all digestive, windy problems
- Stimulate mind and heart so bring joy

Cayenne

- Excellent *adjuvent* (increases effects of other medicines) when coldness or poor circulation
- Tastes very hot and may upset sore mouths or throats
- Speeds up circulation and relaxes artery walls, so promoting blood flow
- Will speed digestion
- Can be used in poultices where warmth required
- Can be used for reviving people subsequent to heart attacks

Celery

- Diuretic and excretor of uric acid, therefore good cleanser and used in gout, rheumatism or when gentle cleansing required
- Seeds more powerful than stalks
- Good source of calcium

strengthener, will help weak constitutions
- Can be used in poultices for arthritis

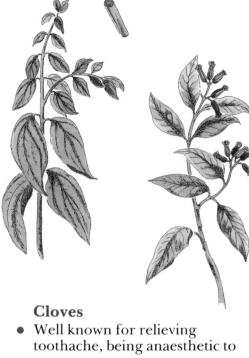

Cloves

- Well known for relieving toothache, being anaesthetic to gums
- Oil applied to back will help kidney energy, so useful if lacking lustre
- Disinfectant effect acts upon lungs and lymphatics

Coriander

- Digestive, relieving digestive spasms, wind build-up, bad breath
- Seeds stimulate gastric juices, reduce phlegm production
- Effective in reducing allergic

Chicory

- Gentle liver stimulant
- Helps relieve constipation
- Helps blood sugar problems, such as diabetes, hypoglycaemia

Cinnamon

- Warming, will stop colds and flu developing
- An excellent digestive
- A circulatory stimulant and

reactions, such as hayfever, rashes
- Use externally for arthritis and to stop bleeding

Cucumber
- Cooling, cleansing, diuretic so will help hot, inflamed conditions when eaten or used directly on the skin

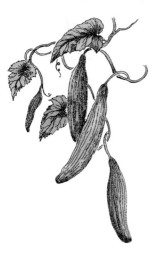

Dill
- Dispels wind, digestive

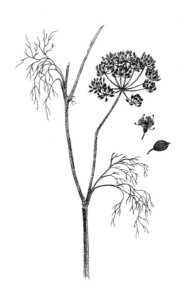

Fennel seed
- Speeds slow digestion
- Helps fat digestion, reducing build-up of wind
- Encourages milk production
- Diuretic, will help some urinary problems

Cumin
- Digestive tonic, eases flatulence, hiccups, belching

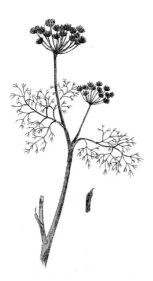

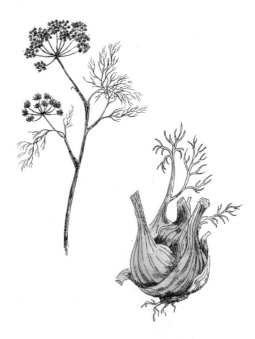

Fenugreek

- Used for convalescence, debility
- A nerve tonic

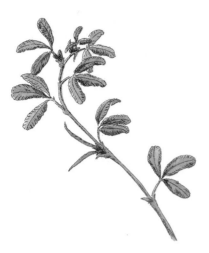

Figs

- Laxative, soothing, very good for constipation
- Soothe inflammation
- High in vitamins, minerals
- High sugar content, so avoid in diabetes

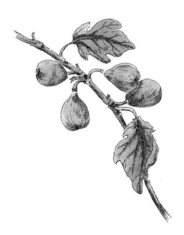

Garlic

- Antibiotic yet spares friendly bacteria in digestive and respiratory tract so aids treatments for bronchitis, colds, candida and other infections
- Excellent for lowering cholesterol
- Can worsen some complaints such as psoriasis, and aggravate a stomach ulcer

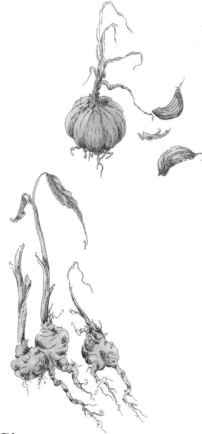

Ginger

- Warming plant encouraging blood to the periphery (hands, feet, skin)
- Tonic to the respiratory tract
- Warms stomach, aiding digestion and reducing nausea, therefore excellent for travel sickness
- Include in remedies for flatulence, colds, wherever gentle warming required
- Dried ginger generally more effective than fresh

Honey

- Healing, antiseptic, antibiotic
- Can be applied to burns
- Used in making herbal syrups
- Soothing for sore throats. Combines well with lemon

Lemon

- Antiseptic juice high in vitamin C
- Neutralises acidity in body
- Can be applied to boils, acne, eczema, sinus congestion, dandruff
- Useful for liver problems, colds, coughs, sore throats

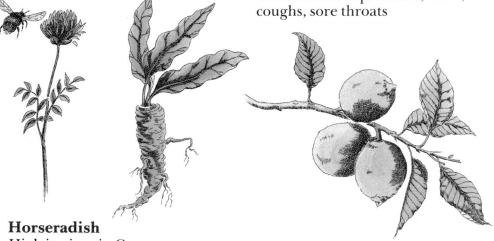

Horseradish

- High in vitamin C
- Antibiotic
- Good circulatory stimulant
- Promotes healing
- Stimulates stomach secretions
- A solvent of excess mucus
- Reduces hayfever symptoms
- Can cause blisters when applied directly to skin

Juniper

- Urinary tract antiseptic
- Diuretic
- Must not be used in pregnancy

Marjoram (sweet or pot)

- Expectorant, antiseptic, carminative, antispasmodic
- Accelerates healing by increasing white blood cell count
- Useful for digestive disorders where tension but lack of energy
- Relaxing tonic

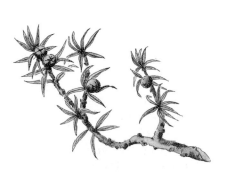

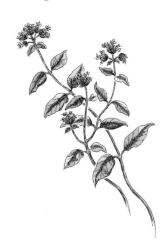

Mint

- Excellent after-dinner digestive
- Reduces nausea, colic, wind
- Mild painkiller
- Oil eases itchy rashes, such as chickenpox, and speeds recovery of most viral illnesses

Nutmeg

- Warm, bitter, digestive
- Eases bloating, windy conditions
- Increases absorption from small intestine
- Has calming effect and can induce sleep

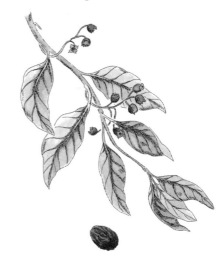

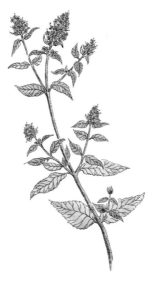

Mustard

- Used for centuries in hand and foot baths to stop colds, chills developing
- Speeds up slow digestion

Onions

- Anti-infective, stimulant, tonic, especially to lungs and digestive system
- Use syrup for colds
- Use raw on boils
- Boiled sliver in ear overnight reduces earache

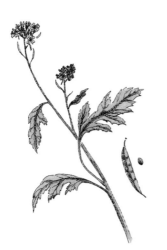

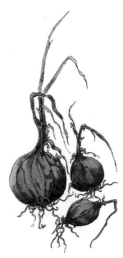

Oregano

- Clears respiratory and genito-urinary infections
- Aids digestion

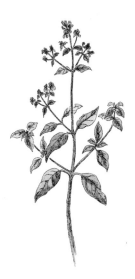

Pepper

- Hot, can be used like chilli to stimulate circulation
- Expectorant

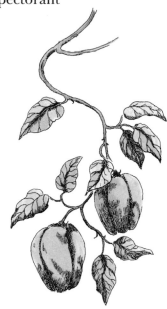

Parsley

- Most beneficial for anaemia sufferers due to high iron, vitamin, mineral content
- Diuretic, cleansing, stimulates bile production
- Relieves build-up of fluid

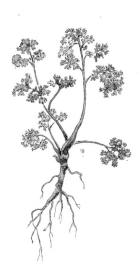

Rosemary

- Warming
- Stimulates circulation, especially to brain, bringing greater awareness, aiding memory, lifting depression
- Stimulates the liver

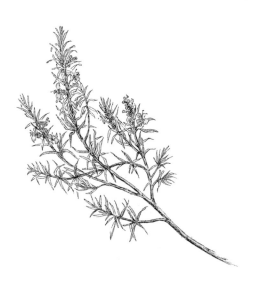

Sage

- Antibiotic, astringent, so a good mouthwash, gargle, poultice for sore mouths and throats
- Contains oestrogen-like substances and reduces sweating, so widely used in menopausal problems
- Dries up milk production, excess mucus

Tarragon

- Digestive
- Calms nervous agitation
- Useful in calming today's stressed digestive systems

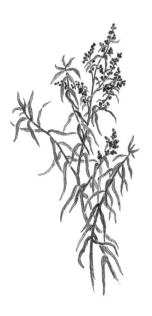

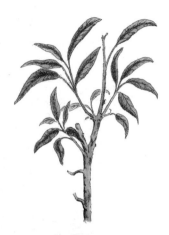

Savory

- Adrenal tonic, stimulant, digestive, antiseptic
- Increases general vitality

Thyme

- Warming, toning, antiseptic, expectorant
- Highly antiseptic
- Excellent for clearing infections, especially chest, bowel, urinary tract

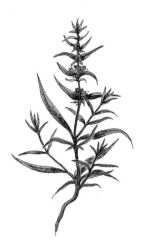

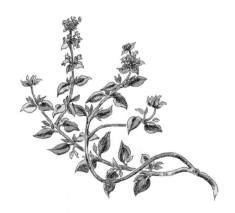

8

HERBAL FIRST AID

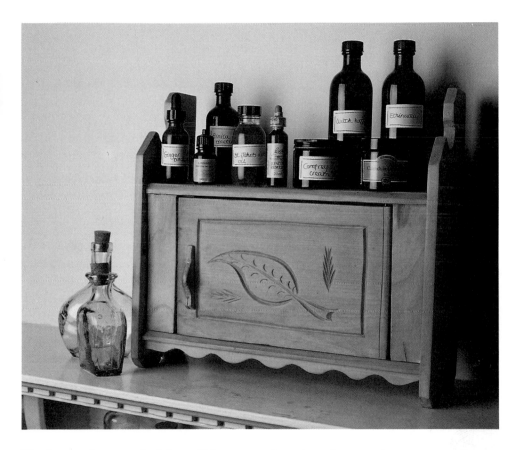

Herbs work remarkably well in acute situations but we suggest you also do a first aid course to learn resuscitation, the recovery position, how to deal with amputations, choking and other emergencies.

Burns

- Put the burnt area under cold water immediately and keep it there for a few minutes.

- Apply **St John's wort oil**, **lavender essential oil**, **calendula cream** or **aloe gel** every hour.

- If the burns are severe, you must seek hospital treatment immediately.

Broken bones, fractures

- Obviously hospital treatment is essential but the healing can be greatly speeded up by using **comfrey leaf** as a tea, 1 tsp per cup 3 times a day for up to 8 weeks.

- If you have ready access to the area, that is, no plaster in the way, use **comfrey cream** daily, with some **cayenne tincture** added to it if possible, 10 ml per 60 ml of cream.

Bruises

- If you bruise easily, find out if it is because you are vitamin K deficient or if you simply have weak capillaries.

- If the bruising occurs for no apparent reason, and you do not normally bruise easily, seek professional advice.

- Apply **horsechestnut**, **witch hazel** (the distilled variety is less astringent), or **arnica**, as lotion or cream. **Comfrey** ointment is an ideal healing base.

Cuts and grazes

- Seek medical attention if wounds are deep or gaping.

- Clean area with diluted tincture of **calendula**, **myrrh** or **golden seal**.

- Use **witch hazel**, **St John's wort**, **lavender** or **comfrey** as healing agents, as creams, oils, teas or lotions dabbed over the area.

Insect bites

- If you are sensitive to bites you can take herbs to prevent over-reactions. See *Allergies*.

- It is possible to take plants to make your skin smell repellent to insects but be unnoticeable to us.

- Apply repellants, such as **rosemary**, **lavender**, **tea tree**, **lemon grass** or **citronella** to you or your clothes.

- Alternatively take **feverfew** – 10 drops of tincture, 2 tablets or 2 leaves twice a day.

- Hang a bunch of **rue**, **rosemary**, **tansy**, **southernwood** and **wormwood** in your room for a similar effect.

- Tinctures of **St John's wort**, **curled dock**, **arnica**, **feverfew** and **witch hazel** mixed equally with **essential oils of lavender**, **tea tree** ease the irritation and prevent infection.

- If you are strongly allergic to stings, it is wise to keep **ephedra** on hand to take while you go for medical attention.

- Dab on essential oil of **lavender** or cold, distilled **witch hazel** to soothe itching bites.

Nose bleeds

- Ensure that high blood pressure is not the cause.

- Seek medical attention if the nose bleed follows a blow to the head.

- Apply cold compresses of **witch**

hazel or **yarrow** to the back of the neck.

Shock

- The best known remedy for shock, usually resulting from a fall, accident or bad news, is the **Bach flower rescue remedy**, which is easily available and easy to use.

- Alternatively use no more than 3 drops of **arnica** tincture in a glass of water.

Splinters

- Draw splinters out with an ointment consisting of **marshmallow root** and **slippery elm bark**.

- Powder the roots and add to any base or innocuous cream.

Sprains

- Immediately apply ice or cold water to the area to reduce the swelling.

- Dab on **arnica** or **witch hazel**. This reduces the amount of bruising.

- Drink **comfrey leaf** to speed the healing. Then apply **comfrey cream**, ideally with **cayenne tincture** added to increase the blood flow in the area.

- If you can do nothing else, crushed cabbage leaves applied to the area will hasten recovery.

Sunburn

- Apply **aloe vera gel** or **St John's wort oil** to the skin.

- Distilled **witch hazel** is soothing.

Toothache

- **Oil of clove** is the traditional remedy and works exceptionally well, although it makes you salivate profusely.

- If the pain is due to an abscess, use **poke root** and **echinacea**, obtained from a herbalist.

Travel sickness

- To avoid travel sickness take 10 drops of **ginger tincture** 10 minutes or so before setting off by car, boat or plane.

- Seabands which you put around your wrist are available from major chemists. They have a little plastic knob that presses on an acupuncture point to relieve nausea.

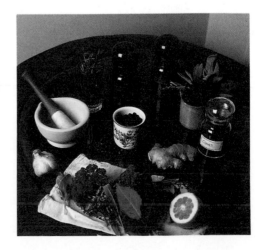

FURTHER READING

Barnard, Julian and Martine, *The Healing Herbs of Edward Bach*, Bach
  Educational Programme, 1988
Campion, Kitty, *Woman's Herbal*, Vermilion, 1992
Chaitow, Leon, *Vaccination and Immunization*, C.W. Daniel, 1987
Elliot, Rose and De Paoli, Carlo, *Kitchen Pharmacy*, Chapmans, 1991
Grant, Doris and Joice, Jean, *Food Combining for Health*, Thorsons, 1991
Grieve, M., *A Modern Herbal*, Penguin Books, 1980
Griggs, Barbara, *Green Pharmacy*, Jill Norman & Hobhouse, 1982
Kenton, Leslie and Susannah, *Raw Energy*, Arrow Books, 1989
Kitzinger, Sheila, *Freedom and Choice in Childbirth*, Penguin, Books, 1988
McIntyre, Anne, *The Herbal for Mother and Child*, Element Books, 1992
McIntyre, Michael, *Herbal Medicine for Everyone*, Penguin Books, 1990
Mills, Simon, *A–Z of Modern Herbalism*, Thorsons, 1989
Schauenberg, Paul and Paris, Ferdinand, *Guide to Medicinal Plants*,
  Lutterworth Press, 1990
Weiss, Rudolf Fritz, *Herbal Medicine*, Arcanum, 1988

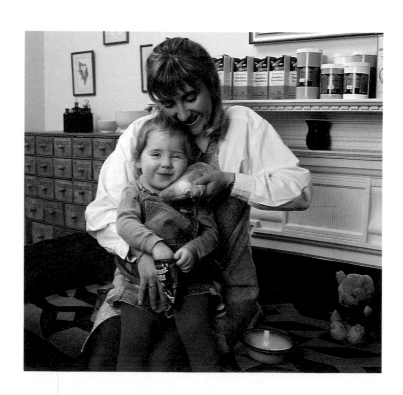

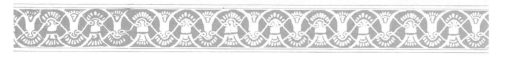

USEFUL ADDRESSES

National bodies

National Institute of Medical Herbalists
9 Palace Gate
Devon EX1 1JA
(*contact for directory of qualified herbalists*)

The British Herbal
Medicine Association
The Old Coach House
Southborough Road
Surbiton
Surrey

The Herb Society
77 Great Peter Street
London SW1

The Healthy House
Cold Harbour
Ruscombe
Stroud
Gloucestershire GL6 4DA
(Tel: 0453-752216)

National Childbirth Trust
Alexandra House
Oldham Terrace
London W3 6NH

Active Birth Centre
55 Dartmouth Park Road
London NW5

The Women's
Environmental Network
Information Officer
WEN Trust
Aberdeen Studios
22 Highbury Grove
London N5 2EA

Training and courses

The School of Phytotherapy (Herbal
Medicine)
Bucksteep Manor
Bodle Street Green
Hailsham
East Sussex
(Tel: 0323-833812)
(*offer the only full-time course*)

Scottish School of Herbal Medicine
PO Box 52
Glasgow G4 0OT

Dr Christopher's School of
Natural Healing
19 Park Terrace
Stoke-on-Trent
Staffordshire ST6 6PB

Herbal suppliers

Arkocaps
Arkopharma
6 Redlands Centre
Redlands
Coulsden
Surrey CR5 2HT

Frances Büning & Paul Hambly
(*authors of this book*)
65 Frant Road
Tunbridge Wells
Kent TN2 5LH
(Tel: 0892-545542)

Baldwins
171/173 Walworth Road
London SE17 1RW
(Tel: 071-703 5550)

Brome & Schimmer
Romsey Industrial Estate
Romsey
Hants SO51 0HR
(Tel: 0794-515595)

East West Herbs
Langston Priory Mews
Kingham
Oxon OX7 6UP
(Tel: 0608-658862)

Gaia Herbal Apothecary
London Road
Forest Row
East Sussex RH18 5EZ
(Tel: 0342-822716)

Gerard House
475 Capability Green
Luton LU1 3LU
(Tel: 0582-487331)

Hambleden Herbs
(*organic herbs*)
16 Ingate Place
London SW8 3NS
(Tel: 071-498 8689)

The Herbal Apothecary
(*many organic herbs*)
103 The High Street
Syston
Leicester LE7 8GQ
(Tel: 0533-602690)

Lanes
Mayflower Road
Plymouth
Devon

Napiers Dispensary
18 Bristo Place
Edinburgh EH1 1EZ
(Tel: 031-225 5542)

Neal's Yard Apothecary
2 Neal's Yard
Covent Garden
London WC2H 9DP
(Tel: 071-371 7662)
(*also around the country*)

Potter's Herbal Supplies
Leyland Mill Lane
Wigan
Lancs WN1 2SB
(Tel: 0942-34761)

Capsules

Davcaps
PO Box 11
Monmouth
Gwent NP5 3NX

East West Herbs
address as above

Hambleden Herbs
(*vegan capsules also*)
address as above

The Herbal Apothecary
(*vegan capsules also*)
address as above

Essential oils

Amphora Aromatics
36 Cotham Hill
Cotham
Bristol BS6 6LA

Gerard House
address as above

The Herbal Apothecary
address as above

Neal's Yard
address as above

Tisserand
Aromatherapy Supplies
The Knoll Business Centre
Old Shoreham Road
Hove
East Sussex
(Tel: 0273-412139)

Food supplements

Biocare
54 Northfield Road
Kings Norton
Birmingham B30 1JH
(Tel: 021-433 3727)

G & G Food Supplies
175 London Road
East Grinstead
West Sussex RH19 1YY
(Tel: 0342-312811)

Natural Flow
Burwash Common
East Sussex TN19 7LX
(Tel: 0435-882482)

Cosmetics

Cornucopia
*address as for The Herbal
Apothecary above*

Cosmetics to Go
29 High Street
Poole
Dorset BH15 1AB
(Freephone: 0800-373366)

Neal's Yard
address as above

Weleda
Heanor Road
Ilkeston
Derbyshire DE7 8DR

Herbal medicine and animals

John Rohrbach (*herbal
veterinary surgeon – referral service*)
Ard-Laggan
Perth Road
Crieff
Perthshire PH7 3EQ
(Tel: 0764-653320)

Equiherbs (*for horses*)
103 The High Street
Syston
Leicester LE7 8GQ
(Tel: 0533-602690)